Menopause and Natural Hormones

Charting Your Course Through Your Change of Life

Daved Rosensweet M.D.

Life Medicine and Healing P.A.

Bonita Springs & Sarasota, Florida

This book has been written and published to provide information and should not be used as a substitute for the recommendations of your health care professional. Because each person and medical situation are unique, the reader is urged to review this information with a qualified health professional. You should not consider the information contained in this text to represent the practice of medicine or to replace consultation with a physician or other qualified healthcare provider.

Published by:

Life Medicine and Healing
1460 Golden Gate Parkway
Naples, Florida 34105
941.430.8624
www.MenopauseandNaturalHormones.com
www.RosensweetMD.com
email: rosensweetmd@earthlink.net

ISBN: 0-9726671-1-3

Printed in the United States of America

Menopause and Natural Hormones

Contents

Contents

Acknowledgements

This book has been a collaboration, and I thank deeply and dearly the many people involved.

Catherine Logan inspired me to mobilize fully for menopause and has been a constant ally. Betsy Cole put in so much elbow grease, hashing out the initial edits in the trenches. Thank you Betsy, you were so helpful, strong and humorous.

Of the many medical friends and allies I have had along the way, Brett Jacques N.D. at AAL Laboratories helped fill in some of the exquisite biochemical details in my knowledge over time, and, makes me laugh uproariously. Pioneers and excellence in the field of female medicine, including John Lee M.D. have made a difference. Pharmacists stand out for their support and superb quality of their work, Tom White RPh , Fred Kinnard RPh, and Ross Heim RPh. So many women have benefited from their excellence as well as that of compounding pharmacists everywhere.

The foundation of all that I understand of menopause comes from so many women patients I have had over the years. Their biggest gift always has been their individual beingness, yet it has been the heat of many a flash that has kept my feet to the fire to get this one right. I also acknowledge the women I have seen who have had breast cancer...always the hurt and the question, if things had been different would they have gotten ill?

Fran Lankford, you dear one, would this have happened without you? Betty Crana, your love makes a difference. Mary Reinhart, Andy Little, Lisa Zembal, Terry McKee, Kim Perkins, Lea Semple, Alan Marsh, Bernie Cunningham,

Christine Meistrich and Joshua Rosensweet: special pearls of support have been given.

Thank you Annabelle Fore, Rebecca Gagnon, Lisa Notter, Nancy Griffith, Paula Rigg, Stephanie McDonald, Gina James, Kathy McDonald: people who are and have been so important, caring and supportive of me and this work on a daily basis. David Perlmutter MD, thank you.

Thank you Bonny Hawley for the beauty and magic of your cover art, and for the generosity of coming forward to offer to create it and then give it as a gift. Thank you.

And Eisa Marshall: thank you for who you are and the gift of making my days go forward with so much caring and brightness.

Shea Lindner, thank you for your hours and hours and hours, and ease, strength and grace. This book would not be, without you. It has been a pleasure and a joy, and I am so grateful for your skill, risks and gifts.

Thanks to Sparkle, Star, Wonder and Carlos for your love and company of Shea and I thoughout the process.

Lazaris' love and support makes an unnameable difference. Thank you Lazaris.

Lyn, your love, wisdom and courage have changed the course of my eternal existence. I love you and am grateful forever. And your chapter (wow!) and other contributions to this book have added to its richness and depth.

Thank you, all of you.

Preface

Shortly before this book was going to its first printing, the stories started exploding onto national news about the dangers of hormonal treatment for menopausal women. This exposure is truly a miracle! For thirty years there have been many doctors and scientists who have raised safety questions about conventional practices in treating women with hormones, especially treating with estrogens derived from horse urine. For the last decade, at least, we have had strong scientific evidence that there are many women who have gotten serious illnesses from the most commonly used of these hormonal products, Premarin and PremPro. For several decades many doctors, pharmacists and other practitioners, as well as women with this concern, have sought to understand this topic and offer better solutions.

The increased incidences of cancer, heart disease, and stroke, seen in the national study with PremPro are not simple issues. It is not accurate to blame the whole of these illnesses on hormones. In this large scientific study, the incidence of breast cancer was increased in women who were treated with PremPro, as compared to women who did not receive this treatment. This increase of incidence is shocking and tragic, and the study was abandoned. Among many things that can be said, it is a miracle in America that diligence and a free press can lead to massive exposure of wrongness in a New York minute. Also to be considered is that the vast majority of women being treated did not get breast cancer. Certainly the women that did get ill had other vulnerabilities and frailties related to immune system, toxicity, nutrition and stress, all of which play a fundamental role in the development of any life-threatening illness.

It will not be good enough to conclude that hormones are bad and should never be used. The symptoms from hormone deficiency are no picnic, and, these deficiencies are often detrimental for health. Behind the abandoned PremPro study, was the strong suspicion that hormones could make a beneficial difference for heart and bones. Many women with severe symptoms and many doctors who treat menopausal women know that simply stopping all treatment with hormones will not fly.

Hormones, like any remedy, can be used impeccably or, can be abused. Elegance and safety can be increased with scrupulous care to discover the details of the individual woman, with regards to risk factors, hormonal needs, balance and dosages. It should be emphasized that it is of the utmost importance to use natural, molecularly-identical hormones prepared by 'compounding' pharmacists. Also important is for each individual woman to be an active participant in the determination of her optimal dosages.

We understand a great deal about what puts a woman at risk for severe illness and, with care and effort, these details can be evaluated and minimized. Again, there are so many other factors that determine increased risk for severe illness. As far as risk relates to hormones, the hormones of concern are the estrogens. This large scientific study involving PremPro had many problems: horse derived genotoxic estrogens, one-dose-fits-all, and failure to evaluate and eliminate from this study women at significant risk. It is time to end, among these other issues, the use of horse-derived estrogens and remove these from the market.

Even when using natural estrogens under the most ideal

and refined of programs, we are not quite able to guarantee safety. We do not have sufficient experience with long term impeccable usage of natural estrogens, nor do we have information collected via scientific studies. So we offer this book as a guideline to the details that can help each individual woman make the wisest, safest and most empowered choices possible.

In approaching menopause, it is time to discover that every single individual woman's situation needs to be evaluated in significant detail for needs, risks, benefits, safety and personal preferences. At this time in history it is optimal for each woman, to the best of her ability, to become sufficiently informed on the whole topic to be an active, aggressive, and knowledgeable participant in her own program. It is ideal for those whose situation seems favorable and safe, to use natural molecularly-identical hormones, and to discover, through trial, individually tailored dosage levels; no less, and certainly, no more than is optimal.

This book is about knowledge, individualizing, optimal treatment, natural hormones and multidimensional issues. This book is about making menopause as absolutely safe and elegant as possible.

Chapter One

Menopause: An Elegant Experience

Menopause changes your life. You will never be the same again. Menopause can be a smooth journey for some women and a rocky road for others. For all, there is the possibility of new dimensions of love and joy.

Women, at times, may experience menopause to be uncomfortable or unhealthy, and may choose to seek treatment. Hormonal treatment has been extremely common for decades, and the most commonly prescribed hormones for menopause have been animal derived and genotoxic. They can be dangerous. There *are* other methods of treatment. For one thing, naturally derived bio-identical hormones are available.

There are fundamental principles of treatment I hold as essential. Committed attention to the biological details of you as an individual, and the whole process of menopause is the first. It is crucial to assess all possible choices in the context of your personal risk factors. And, to treat menopause elegantly, it is essential to go beyond hormones and include the rest of your body and your life. This book is about treating menopause elegantly.

Menopause changes your life

You may be troubled by symptoms, such as sleep disturbance, hot flashes, emotional instability, weight gain, bone loss, low energy and difficulties in relationships and life. You may be concerned about risk for heart and female organ disease, hip fracture, and other problems. Hormonal deficiencies and imbalances can underlie many of these issues. It is a great time to pause and consider all of this. It's a time in life to pause and heal.

You can find and choose something different. Begin by learning about menopause, and becoming empowered from your learning. Continue by being one of the most important participants in identifying your personal hormonal needs, making choices in the context of your overall health and specific risk factors, choosing natural bio-identical hormones when hormones are appropriate, and discovering your right dosages and balance. This book is about learning, discovering, identifying and choosing.

In my thirty-two years of practice as a medical doctor I am grateful and excited to be treating women in a time when we have a much more thorough understanding of menopause. The human body is so complex, intricate, amazing and miraculous! Today we have a far more extensive knowledge of the biology of the body than ever before.

Menopause involves hormonal issues. Hormonal products are now available to you that are molecularly identical to hormones produced in your ovaries, and, are derived from natural sources. High-resolution testing is also obtainable, when needed, that can focus in on your individual hormonal picture, and help define aspects of risk.

Years ago, I did not have the same enthusiasm about being able to help women in menopause. Understanding was limited. Also, treatment protocols and products being used were of questionable safety and effectiveness.

Safety: Primum Non Nocere, Do No Harm!

Safety is a key issue and the highest priority in the treatment of menopause. Hormones are involved and hormones are potent. They are beneficial when used with care, expertise and accuracy, and harmful when not.

Forty years ago the incidence of severe female-related illnesses was so much less than it is today. Hormones are a part of this deterioration. When I was in medical school in the mid 1960's breast cancer was a rare disease. This is not so now. I have worked with women, even in their late thirties, who have had breast cancer and it is tragic! At times, their medical history reveals obvious suggestions of hormonal overload, imbalance, even toxicity, or aggravation by hormones and toxins found in the food supply. I have witnessed so many incidences of incorrect prescription of hormonally active medications, including, in some cases, birth control pills. There is more to an illness so profound as cancer than just hormones. Yet, hormones can play a role. Knowing what we know now and paying attention to details can avert so much of this tragedy.

Many women avoid taking hormones because of safety concerns, even though reduced levels of their ovarian hormones are causing personal discomfort or even impairment of their health and well-being. All of the safety issues call for an examination of the multitude of details and risk factors pertaining to the uniqueness of each woman. The ability to make safe choices derives from a thorough knowledge of the individual woman as well as prescription of the safest hormones available.

A wonderful thing about this time in history is that we know enough details about the process of menopause and the causes of illness. We have safe enough and good enough hormones to utilize. The knowledge and tools exist. However, it does require a willingness to individualize each woman's situation. Because of the complexity, this can take real care and effort. A remarkable thing is that with diligence, attention to details, and at times, unravelling issues that go beyond hormones, awesome and safe things can be accomplished. You can be a most significant determiner of that success and that safety. This book is about bringing as much safety to this process as possible. This book is about you taking as much responsibility for that safety as is possible.

Why Treat Menopause?

In addition to the biological factors in menopause that you may face, there can be challenges in your relationships, jobs, and other core life issues. Hormones can dramatically affect your mood, energy, vitality and sexuality. If you do not successfully treat the biologic issues of menopause, you may have more difficulty resolving the other issues in your life. With unbalanced and insufficient hormones you could be operating out of tiredness rather than vitality, sleep deprivation rather than being rested, mood swings rather than emotional stability, and even disease rather than health. Emotions, mind, life, and body are all interwoven. The stress from unresolved issues of life can result in significant glandular fatigue, and then further hormonal reduction and imbalance. All of this can compound physical hardship!

I can picture specific women in menopause who have

come to me in emotional crisis. These were strong women with good lives, and they were in breakdown! They insisted that I forget about how I had known them to be and wanted me to carefully attend to the horribleness of how they felt. To our delight, careful evaluation and right treatment got them back into life with gusto!

I do not want to alarm you and suggest that menopause has to be ever so hard. Many women have passed through menopause with hardly a ruffle! Many women take nothing for menopause. You could also have an easy time. This book is about making menopause as easy as possible.

You could have an easy time of it all

Individuality

Menopause is a biologically complex process in and of itself. Additionally, considerable variations exist from woman to woman in hormone levels, hormone balance, biologic individuality, and general health. The infinite individual variations in body size and biological makeup are natural and of critical importance. Your soul speaks to you through your body. And each individual woman embodies a unique expression of All That Is. This is a magnificence of your soul. Every single face, body type, and shape is needed to express the whole.

Menopause is a biologically complex process with considerable variations existing from woman to woman

Each individual woman embodies a unique expression of the All That Is

Hormones are one of the influences in the development of body type, shape, proportion, and size. In order to manifest this myriad of biological variations, there are as many differences in hormone levels and balance, woman to woman, as there are body sizes and types of women on earth. Of course, hormones are not the only factor that determine body shape: health habits, for example, also play a very significant role.

Every single face, body type, and shape of woman is needed to express the whole.

All of the possible individual differences make the' one-dose-fits-most' approach of commonly prescribed 'hormone replacement therapies' (HRT) hard to figure. There are just too many variations in hormonal balance, woman to woman, to oversimplify dosage to 1 or 2 sizes.

I believe the optimal approach to elegantly treating menopause is for each individual woman to have a significant understanding of the biological process. This includes developing an awareness about how your own individual body works, uncovering and reducing possible personal risk factors related to female organ disease, and making choices

To elegantly treat menopause it is optimal for each individual woman to have a significant understanding of the biological process, along with her individual body and possible risk factors.

for treatment accordingly. It is also crucial, if you choose treatment by hormones, that you use the best quality, combinations and doses of bio-identical hormones. This book is about charting your course, and giving you a roadmap.

Coming up with, and implementing, a strategy about menopause is especially important during perimenopause, the time when a woman's cycle becomes irregular but menstruation is still occurring. During perimenopause hormonal fluctuations can be dramatic and may require that a woman continually adjust her treatment program. During perimenopause, if ovulation ceases, estrogens will overdominate and this is not healthy or even safe. Designing a roadmap and charting a course can be significantly helpful, even before you enter menopause.

It is also of crucial importance to have a kind, understanding, professional practitioner to be a partner in this process and add expert support and guidance along the way. They can often sense or evaluate difficulties that call for specific action. You can benefit most with an experienced professional who listens to you, and what you want and need. Then, together, and with quality information, you can develop a treatment program specifically tailored for you.

When it has come to the practical understanding and application of the biochemistry of hormones by health professionals however, there has been considerable variation and lack of uniformity amongst them. There have been thousands of doctors, pharmacists, and practitioners that, for decades, have identified difficulties with conventional methods of treating menopause. They have researched and found far more thorough, encompassing, and safer methods of evaluation and treatment with hormones. These findings have for the most part, been ignored. There is a lag time in medicine where the best knowledge can take even decades to make it all the way into the mainstream. Impeccable practice has not quite made it to prime time.

I have worked with so many women whose lives have changed dramatically with this approach, which so many practitioners are now presenting. Angie is 53 and had her last period at the age of 40. She is a successful professional, an avid athlete, and married. She had been on a variety of hormones since the onset of menopause yet still had sleep difficulties. She also had a lot lower energy and libido than she was used to. In her treatment, after adequate assessment, we made adjustments in the types and methods of application regarding her hormones. She learned how to find her optimal doses. I did not see her for awhile after this. One day as I was leaving my office, she drove up and jumped out of her car. With great exuberance she exclaimed that she was doing just fabulously again and wanted me to know about her success! She hadn't felt this alive and passionate about her life in a long time.

Menopause can be a challenge worth getting right! If you have heard uncomfortable stories from your friends or on the news, know that you can do it all differently. You can create your own menopause, which does not have to be what you have heard, seen or expect. Your menopause can be addressed carefully, thoroughly, safely, and elegantly. You can do this. So many women have! This book is about learning what, why and how. This book is about success with menopause! This book is about elegance.

You can do it! So many women have.

Chapter Two

Relationship of Menopause to Other Factors

While we may think of menopause biologically as an ovarian hormonal event, it is in fact, so much more. There is a profound physiologic and biochemical interplay. Along with the overlapping within the hormonal system, the intestinal and immune systems, the emotions, and all other systems directly affect menopause.

Biologically, menopause is so much more than an ovarian hormonal event

All of the glands, as pictured in figure 1 on the following page, and all of the glandular hormones are related to one another. As that famous medical song declares, "...the knee bone is connected to the thigh bone, the thigh bone's connected to the hip bone..." When one gland is affected, they all are affected. For example, if we are under stress, we automatically shift into a multidimensional 'fight or flight' mode. The adrenal glands pour out 'stress' hormones. These excess hormones accelerate performance of the heart, muscles, and much more. This dramatic response provides the 'oomph' for moms to lift cars up and off a child.

When the adrenal glands have been overworking for some time during prolonged stress and become fatigued, other glands in the hormonal system come to their aid. For example, during this time of stress, the thyroid gland will increase its production of thyroid hormones. Like the adrenals, thyroid hormones can also augment physical per-figure 1: The Endocrine Glands

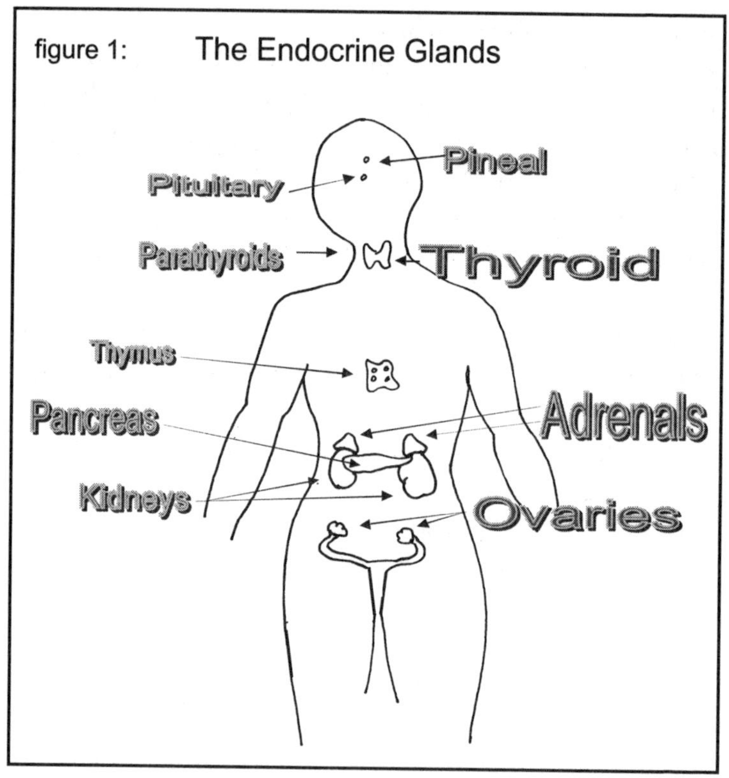

"...the knee bone's connected to the thigh bone, the thigh bone's connected to the hip bone..."

formance, though they do so in a different physiological way. During stress these two glands, the thyroid and adrenals, will rise to the occasion and come to each other's aid for the common good of the whole body.

Ovaries play an integral part in the interrelated glandular system. In times of stress the ovarian/sexual/reproductive system takes a back seat to the high-priority adrenals and thyroid. Stress causes a shift of valuable energy and resources away from the ovaries towards the adrenals and thyroid, leaving the ovaries in a deprived state. The biological consequence of this shift is insufficient production of ovarian hormones.

Ovaries are an integral part of the whole glandular system.

As you can see in figure 2 below, on a biochemical level, the adrenal glands and the ovaries produce many hormones that are related to one another. Most of the hormones, (in general called "steroids"), are derived from a common

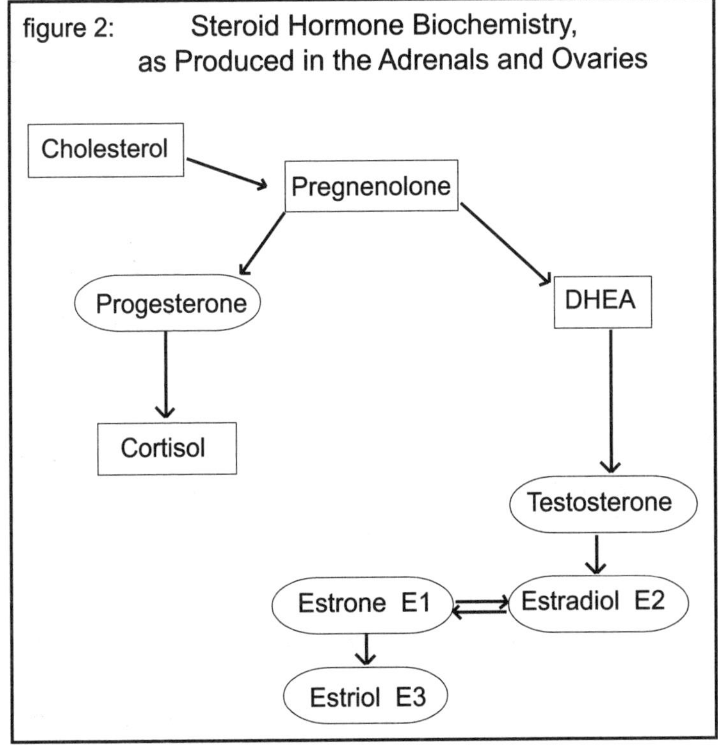

parent hormone called pregnenolone. To understand some fancy biochemistry that occurs during stress, we will follow two hormones: cortisol and the estrogens. When stress occurs, there is an increased need for hormones: the need for cortisol is paramount. Increasing cortisol brings power to the biological stress response. Cortisol is the priority amongst the steroid hormones during stress. Some of the pregnenolone that was destined to become estrogen can be re-routed to add to cortisol production.

You can see the push and pull our hormonal system finds itself in, when functioning in stress mode. It becomes clear why so many women have difficulty with periods during times of stress: their production of ovarian hormones has diminished in favor of the need for increased cortisol. Diminished ovarian hormones will affect timing, amount, and/or symptoms of menstruation. The interconnections of the ovaries with the whole glandular/hormonal system are significant and intimate.

In times of stress the ovarian/sexual/reproductive system takes a back seat to the higher-priority adrenals and thyroid.

There are many instances where we just can't get menopause right until we correct adrenal or thyroid hormone issues. I am thinking now of Jean who was in menopause. She had common symptoms, as well as having a deep fatigue and depression. Her symptoms were only partially alleviated by taking ovarian hormones. When we tested her we found her to be low in thyroid hormone. She improved dramatically when we responded to the thyroid issue in addition to ovarian hormonal imbalances.

Another example of the interrelationship of the hormonal system to other systems occurs with the gastrointestinal system. The intestine, involved with diet, digestion and absorption, is the entry way for the raw materials that make hormones. If intestinal function falters, there will be less nutrients available for hormone production. Because of the greatly diminished amount of cholesterol, the foundation of sex hormones, in vegetarian diets, strict vegetarians can have up to 40% less ovarian hormones than non-vegetarians. Moreover, intestinal function can be adversely affected by infection which is far more common in North America than we used to encounter.

A further interrelationship is seen with the immune system. The immune system requires significant energy and resources to fight viral or occult intestinal infections. In order to do this, the immune system may need to take energy from other sources within the body, like the glandular system for example. This diversion of energy and resources from the glandular to the immune system can ultimately account for reduced glandular function.

There are significant inter-relationships of the hormonal system with the intestinal, immune and other systems.

Alice is a classic example of this. She had chronic fatigue and fibro-myalgia, as well as another illness, for many years. She went into menopause at the age of 36. These illnesses, which included chronic infections, drained energy away from the ovaries, enough to precipitate an early menopause.

Menopause becomes ruthless if the energy and materials have been drawn away from ovarian, sexual and other glandular hormone production. Frequently, to treat menopause successfully, we need to attend to other health issues that pertain to the remainder of the glandular system, and also to the intestinal, immune, and other systems.

Menopause is a complex process. It requires time and dedication to arrive at a safe, reliable, individualized and effective program. The ability to fashion a safer and more precise menopausal strategy has never been as possible as it is now. I encourage you to focus on the fine points, in order to engage in the discovery of your optimal program.

To treat menopause successfully, we frequently need to attend to other body systems and issues.

In light of all this complexity, it is also true that many women have a very easy time in menopause. Ultimately this information is about making your tailored menopausal program as easy as possible.

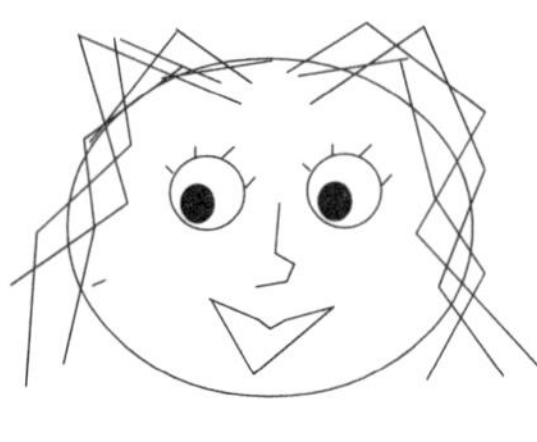

Wow!

Chapter Three

Understanding Menopause

Your Hormonal History

To understand your individual situation and optimal needs, it is valuable to review your own female hormone history. Within that story you will have clues to the balance that has played out in your menstrual life among the hormones produced by your ovaries: the estrogens, progesterone and testosterone. During menopause your body tends to favor and prefer a treatment program that provides a hormonal balance similar to the balance you have experienced in your past.

For example, if you were used to relatively high levels of estrogen during your menstrual years, you probably will not do well in menopause if your estrogen levels sink excessively low. In your case you might enjoy life more by supplementing with natural estrogens. On the other hand, if you had a history of low estrogens and in menopause still produce a decent amount of estrogens in your body fat (this does occur!), supplementing estrogens may not be advisable. Also, supplementing estrogens would not make any sense for a woman at substantial risk for an illness of breast, uterus or ovaries. Further on in this book, as you learn more about the characteristics of the individual hormones and their effects, you will be able to evaluate your earlier hormonal balance.

The Menstrual Cycle

To understand menopause and your hormonal past, we

need first to understand the menstrual cycle itself. The first day of menstrual flow is designated as day one of the menstrual cycle, as depicted in figure 3 below.

In looking at the menstrual cycle, we are going to follow two hormones, estradiol (one of the principle estrogens), and progesterone. During the time of actual menstrual flow, estradiol is present at low levels, and progesterone is present at even lower levels. Estradiol is produced

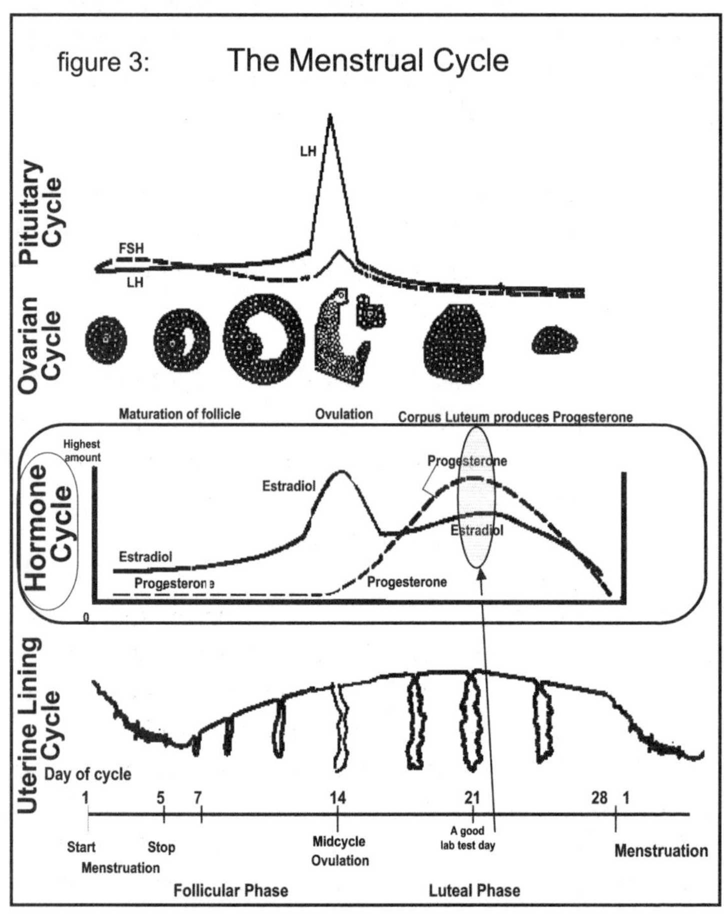

by specific cells in the ovary. Most progesterone is produced by other cells in the ovary: the cells that surround the egg that is ovulated during a cycle.

Hormones made by the pituitary gland also affect the ovaries. In the beginning of the cycle, the pituitary gland produces 'follicle stimulating hormone', commonly called "FSH." This encourages the maturation of one of the thousands of eggs present in the ovaries. The egg that is going to be ovulated turns into a "follicle" and matures further. During this time, the rising estradiol level stimulates development of the lining of the uterus, thus preparing it for possible reception of a fertilized egg.

At midcycle, day 14, there is a surge of the pituitary 'luteinizing hormone,' "LH," and ovulation--the release of the mature ovum or egg-- occurs. Estrogen production, by ovarian cells, peaks at this time.

In the second half of the menstrual cycle, the cells that once surrounded the ovulated egg become known as a "corpus luteum." As a corpus luteum, these cells now turn into a progesterone-producing factory, and levels of progesterone rise dramatically during this time.

If the released egg becomes fertilized by sperm, and then implants in the uterine lining, the lining will mature even further. However, if there is no implantation of a fertilized egg, progesterone levels eventually begin to plummet. This fall in progesterone triggers the shedding of the uterine lining, and menstrual flow begins once again. Pause and think about the extraordinary orchestration of these hormones during the menstrual cycle! The physiology of the pituitary gland, ovary, and the uterus is a miraculous and beautiful symphony.

Estrogen and progesterone, the ovarian hormones that relate to the menstrual cycle, have many other functions. Estrogens stimulate. Estrogens stimulate breast glandular tissue and uterine lining production. Progesterone on the other hand, balances, softens and ameliorates the effects of estrogen. Progesterone supports gestation or pregnancy (hence "pro-gest-ational") and also supports the second half of the menstrual cycle, during which time implantation and initial growth of the fertilized egg can occur.

Estrogens stimulate

Progesterone balances, softens and ameliorates the effects of estrogen

These two hormones are designed to work in harmony. Though we will talk about testing later, note that in figure 3, three-quarters of the way through the menstrual cycle, approximately on day 21, which is half way between ovulation and menstruation, there is a simultaneous peak of both estrogen and progesterone production. This is the ideal time during a cycle to test for these hormones if a woman is still menstruating.

Ponder all of this for a moment: what is going on here? Yikes! I mean, who invented this? Who conceived of it? It's rather awesome when you think and feel about it. And it took place (or still is) in your body!

Think of the extraordinary orchestration of these hormones during the menstrual cycle!

There are many possible variations in the menstrual cycle. The most common duration is 28 days, the same period as the cycle of the moon (think of that!) There are variations possible in cycle length, timing of ovulation, and amount of menstrual flow. The relative amount and balance of the hormones often determine these variations. For example, in figure 4 below, I illustrate a deviation from normal that is quite common: when ovulation does not occur. When this happens, no corpus luteum is formed; there-

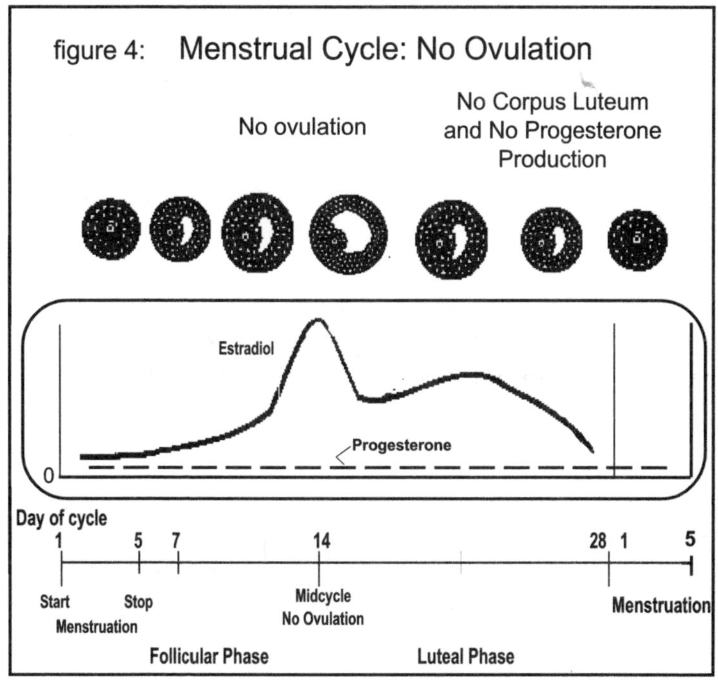

fore there is no significant production of progesterone. In this case, because there is no progesterone to balance the estrogens, the effects on your body, from estrogens, become 'dominant.' In other words, there is simply too much stimulation. Here we have a sneak preview of information that we will detail later: if estrogen stimulation of breast glandular tissue and uterus go unbalanced by progesterone, you can get (or you used to get) breast tenderness, or uterine cramps for example. There even are other more long term changes possible, such as uterine fibroids, or worse!

There are also many other variations of hormonal imbalance in addition to this example of a failure to ovulate.

Just for consideration, ovulation (and thus pregnancy) can occur at any time during a menstrual cycle, even during menstruation.

With a better understanding of the menstrual cycle, we are now ready to learn more about the hormones that drive it.

The most common duration of the menstrual cycle is 28 days, the same period as the cycle of the moon.

Steroid Hormones: Some Basics

There are many systems in the body. The glandular system is one of them. Glands produce hormones. Hormones are potent and have lots of effects. Let's look at some hormones in general and then focus in on the ovarian hormones: estrogens, progesterone and testosterone.

All of the ovarian and testicular hormones and most of the adrenal hormones are closely related biochemically. Most are derived from cholesterol, as I have illustrated in figure 2 (repeated on page 23 for convenience). Cholesterol, which has become a popular household word, is the precursor of the hormones known as "steroids." Cholesterol itself is not hormonally active. These steroid hormones play a significant role in the biochemistry of well-being.

Cholesterol is often addressed as being a problem if it is present at excessive levels in the body. However, what we don't hear much about is the set of problems, like depression, that can develop from cholesterol deficiency. Cholesterol-derived steroid hormones contribute to well-being...lack of them results in lack of well-being. If thyroid hormone from your thyroid gland were to get very low you would live, though you would be extremely tired. To further emphasize the significance of a decrease in steroid levels, this is not true for severely decreased cortisol: without it you would die. Cortisol is critical for life itself.

Cholesterol deficiency will result in diminished steroid hormone production. When cholesterol levels fall too low, adequate amounts of the crucial adrenal hormones, which I mentioned earlier, cannot be produced. Lack of adrenal hormones result in our diminished well-being. In the process of lowering cholesterol, popular prescription drugs sometimes go too far and cause cholesterol deficiency. This can, though rarely, have dire consequences, such as depression and worse. There are other causes of cholesterol deficiency, such as a diet that is insufficient in nutrients. Once again, a strict vegetarian diet can result in up to 40% lower steroid hormones than a non-vegetarian diet.

In the first step of the steroid production pathway, cholesterol is converted to pregnenolone. Pregnenolone, becomes the great grandmother hormone, ancestor to all steroid hormones and has active hormonal effects. Interestingly, it was given to Airforce pilots and factory workers during World War II. When pregnenolone was administered, reports showed a definite increase in their energy, acuity of perception, and general well being. At times we will treat someone with this progenitor of the steroids...giving the body an opportunity to shunt it where it wants. (This does not always produce the effects desired, so more often, we recommend taking the particular hormone in question, especially in specific hormone depletion).

A strict vegetarian diet can result in up to 40% lower steroid hormones than a non-vegetarian diet

Referring again to figure 2 pictured on the next page, pregnenolone can convert into progesterone, and from progesterone, cortisol is produced. When pregnenolone is biochemically metabolized in another way, it produces DHEA, then testosterone, and then the estrogens.

There are three main hormones produced in the ovaries: the estrogens, progesterone and testosterone. Once more, the estrogens and progesterone are designed to work in harmony with each other. Estrogens stimulate breast glandular tissue and are important during pregnancy to assist the maturation of the breasts, eventually for lactation. Progesterone quiets the effect of this stimulation. As I mentioned before, women who do not ovulate, and therefore do not have adequate progesterone to balance and complement the estrogen, often develop significant breast tenderness and PMS from over stimulation. Lack of progesterone may also put one at risk for fibrocystic breast prob-

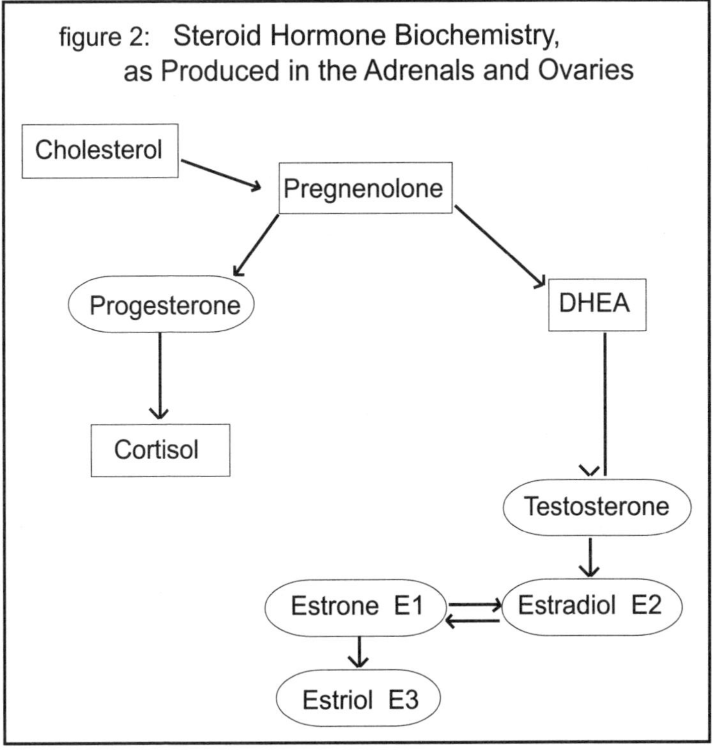

figure 2: Steroid Hormone Biochemistry, as Produced in the Adrenals and Ovaries

lems, endometriosis, uterine diseases and worse.

Looking again at the roadmap in figure 2 on the preceding page, we can see the biochemical detail involved in hormone production. When there is significant stress in our lives, the production of cortisol takes precedence over other hormone pathways. Extra cortisol is needed. Resources are diverted away from the production of the other hormones to produce it. This is known as the "cortisol steal." The "cortisol steal" can ultimately result in diminished levels of the estrogens, testosterone, and progesterone. Stress induced diversion to cortisol wreaks havoc with the menstrual cycle and other ovarian hormone-reliant functions such as libido, mood, and sleep! *One key to helping a younger woman with irregular periods and PMS who may have significant stress, could lie in helping the adrenal glands or the thyroid recover rather than giving her ovarian hormones.* There are other possible issues and resolutions for younger women as well.

Referring once again, to the chart in figure 2, we see that a hormone called DHEA also originates from pregnenolone. As mentioned previously, testosterone is derived from DHEA, and the estrogens are derived from testosterone. Testosterone is a *human* hormone, not just a 'male' hormone. Although men have more than women, testosterone is necessary for both genders. Testosterone has prominent effects on rebuilding metabolism, on the heart and bones, and is one of the principle sustainers of female, as well as male, libido. Individual women differ in the amount of testosterone they are used to and need, just as they differ in the amounts of all other hormones required.

Note that in figure 2, there are three estrogens listed, estrone, estradiol and estriol. Estrone, often abbreviated "E1," and estradiol, "E2," are the most potent of the estrogens. Estriol, "E3," though 'weaker,' is very important for balance with the other two. An illustration of the significance of this balance and the importance of the role ovarian hormones play in health and disease was found in a 1960's medical study designed to uncover any relationship

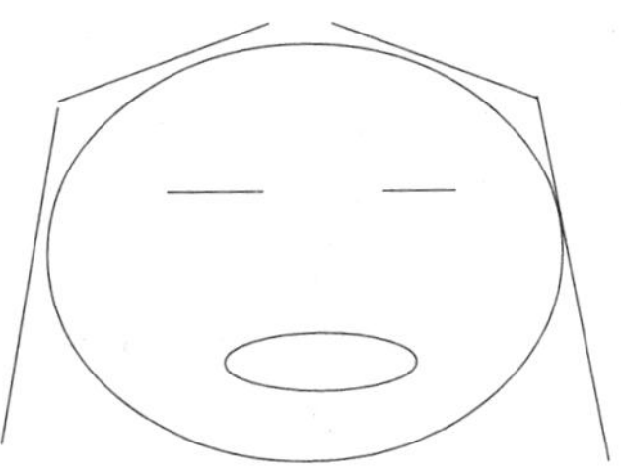

Yikes! This is getting complicated doctor. Why can't you just tell me what to do and keep this medical mumbo jumbo to yourself.

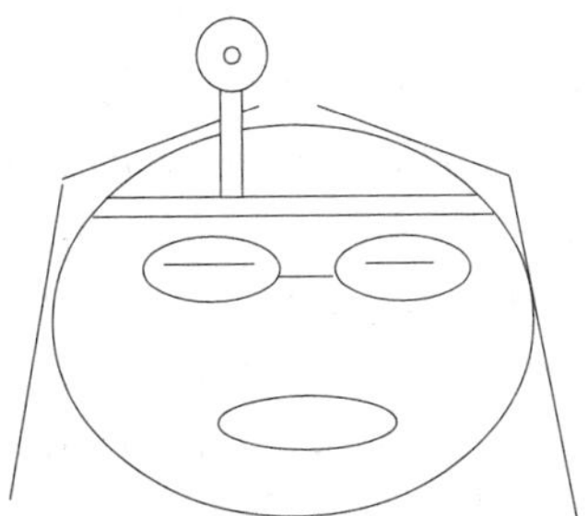

I could Ms Jones. Here's two aspirin. Call me in the morning. Or how about some ether and a biting stick.

between the breast-stimulatory effect of estrogen and breast cancer. Urine samples were collected over a 24-hour period from a group of healthy women, and from another group of women who had breast cancer. When measuring the estrogens, scientists discovered that the healthy women had a much higher percentage of Estriol than the women who had cancer. The balance between these three estrogens is important for health. This balance is biochemically determined by certain nutrients, and processing which takes place in the liver. This study helps us to understand one of the estrogen links to breast cancer. Medical science has unveiled other aspects of this relationship, and we will talk more about this later.

Sarah is a woman who had breast cancer and was four years beyond treatment of it when she came to me for suggestions on how she could prevent recurrence. Among other things, we tested her urine. We found her to have diminished estriol, and through the use of a simple nutrient (diatomic Iodine) were able to restore her estrogens to proper balance with each other.

Chapter Four

Is Menopause, As We Know It, Natural?

I'd like to bring up a challenging question: is menopause, as we currently know it, entirely natural? I bring this up, not to confuse you, but to deepen our understanding. To explore this question, let's begin by looking at hormone levels over time. In figure 5 below, we see that estrogen levels in females begin to rise in the early teens, reach their peak in the late teens or early twenties, and then diminish over time. When those levels diminish enough, menstruation ceases, and we have "menopause."

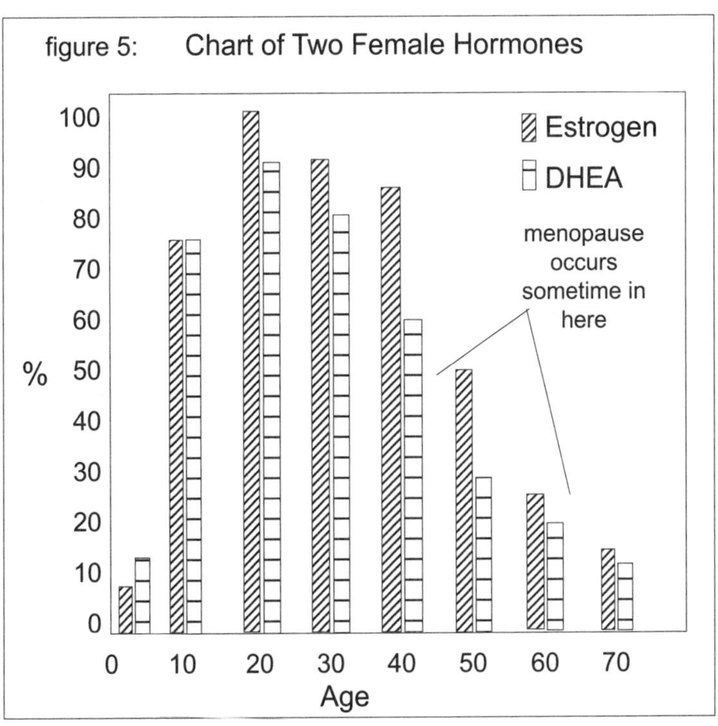

figure 5: Chart of Two Female Hormones

Notice, for comparison, in figure 5 on the preceding page, that a similar pattern of rise and fall occurs with female DHEA levels. DHEA is a hormone not principally produced in the ovary, nor directly related to the menstrual cycle.

Is menopause, as we know it, entirely natural?

One attribute that makes menopause dramatic is that it's a 'threshold' event. In any threshold event, certain processes must take place in order for the event to happen. Menstruation and cycling requires certain ample 'threshold' levels of ovarian hormones to be present. When hormone levels fall beneath a threshold, menstrual cycles and menstruation cease. *It does not matter whether that fall below that threshold is slight or great: once hormone amounts fall beneath a minimum needed to produce an* endometrial lining, *cycling is over.* This cessation is an abrupt and obvious event because it relies on 'threshold' levels. On the other hand, when DHEA declines, changes are not threshold and are gradual and you may or may not notice a lessening of energy and flabbiness developing in your arms.

It is also interesting and remarkable to note in figure 6 on the next page that male hormones follow a similar pattern to the rise and fall of female hormones. Both male DHEA and testosterone levels rise and then decline over time, just as they do in women. We have not been as aware of a major change taking place in men during their midlife as we have been of menopause in women. Obviously males do not have so dramatic an alteration as the cessation of menstruation. When Viagra's popularity revealed that there was an enormous incidence of erectile dysfunction, we were reminded that hormone levels diminish in men as well. The consequences of this decline are profound and go beyond diminishing libido and erection to include effects on mood, stamina, heart, and rejuvenation metabolism.

The point is that all hormone levels in all women and all men, rise then decline over time. I pose this question: is this decline natural?

The charts in figures 5 and 6 represent an average rate of hormonal decline. As you can see in the chart in figure

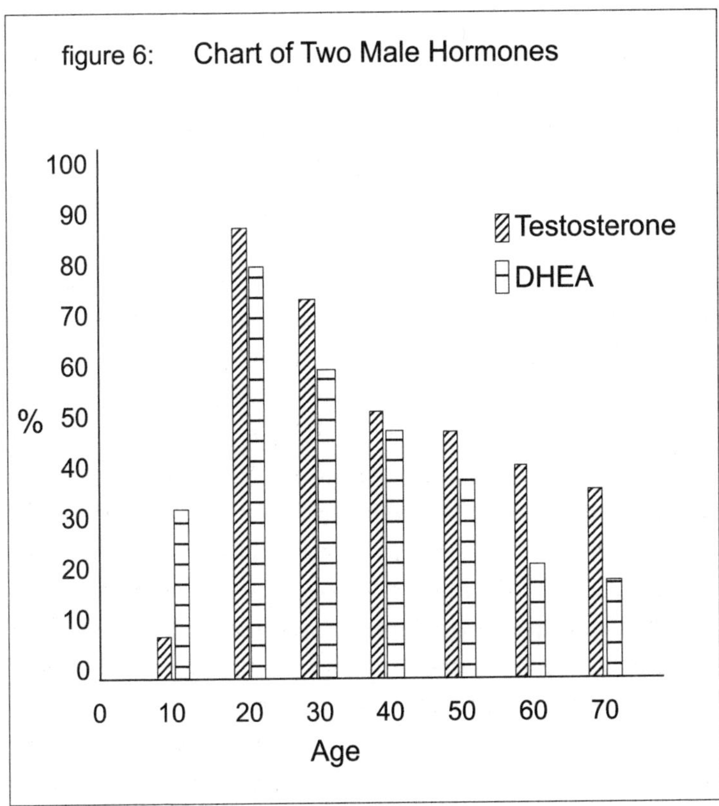

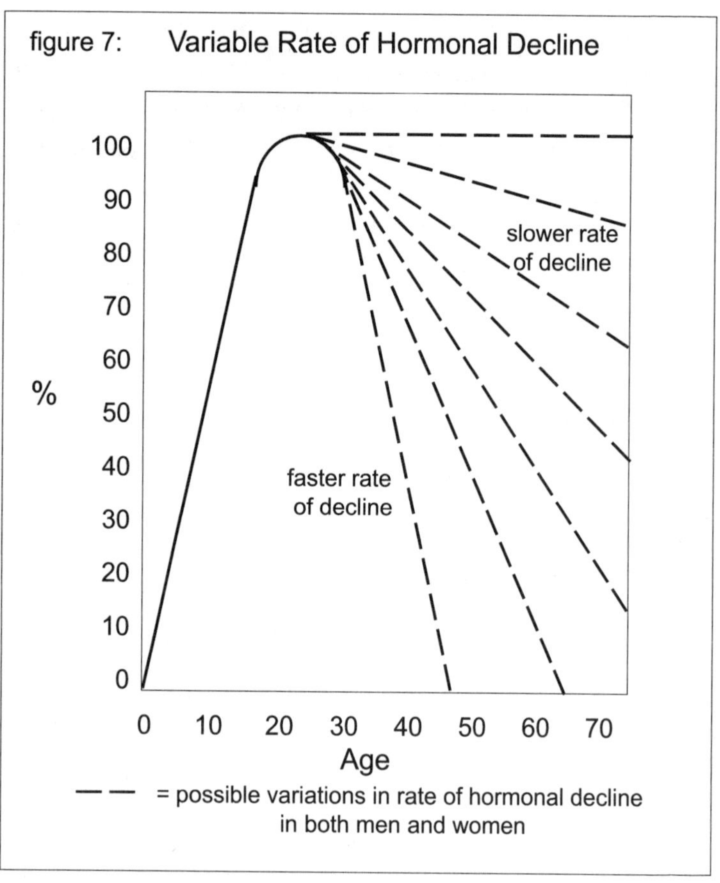

7 above, some women and men have a faster rate of hormonal diminution and wind up with less of these hormones at an earlier age. In others, hormones diminish at a more gradual rate and these people have more hormones at a later age in life. Most women and men notice that they do not have the same hormone levels at age 50 that they had at age 20.

Perhaps we can get more insight into the question, "Is

menopause natural?" by examining when menopause begins. Hormone levels actually begin to decline in our late twenties. Does menopause begin in our twenties, when these hormone levels start to decline? Why do we assume that menopause begins with the cessation of menstruation? Cessation of menstruation is just one bump in the road in the ongoing process of aging or senescence. It's an unusual bump in women because a threshold has been crossed so that changes are dramatic.

All hormone levels in all women and all men rise then decline over time.

As an aside, when can you celebrate no longer needing contraception? The best information that I have came through a personal communication that suggested that you are not completely 'safe' until a year after cessation of periods.

The biggest factor that plays into the question of menopause being natural or not relates to the most profound affector of hormones, described by that 20th and 21st century household word, that unreal phenomenon that appears to be ever-so-real, that phantom, that illusion, presenting the biggest adversity to your hormones. You guessed it! *"Stress!"*

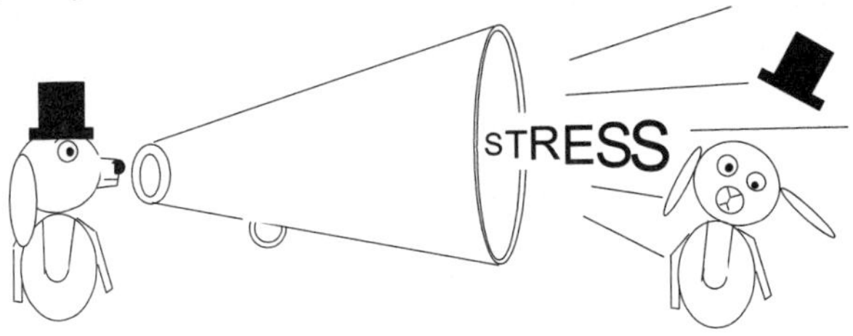

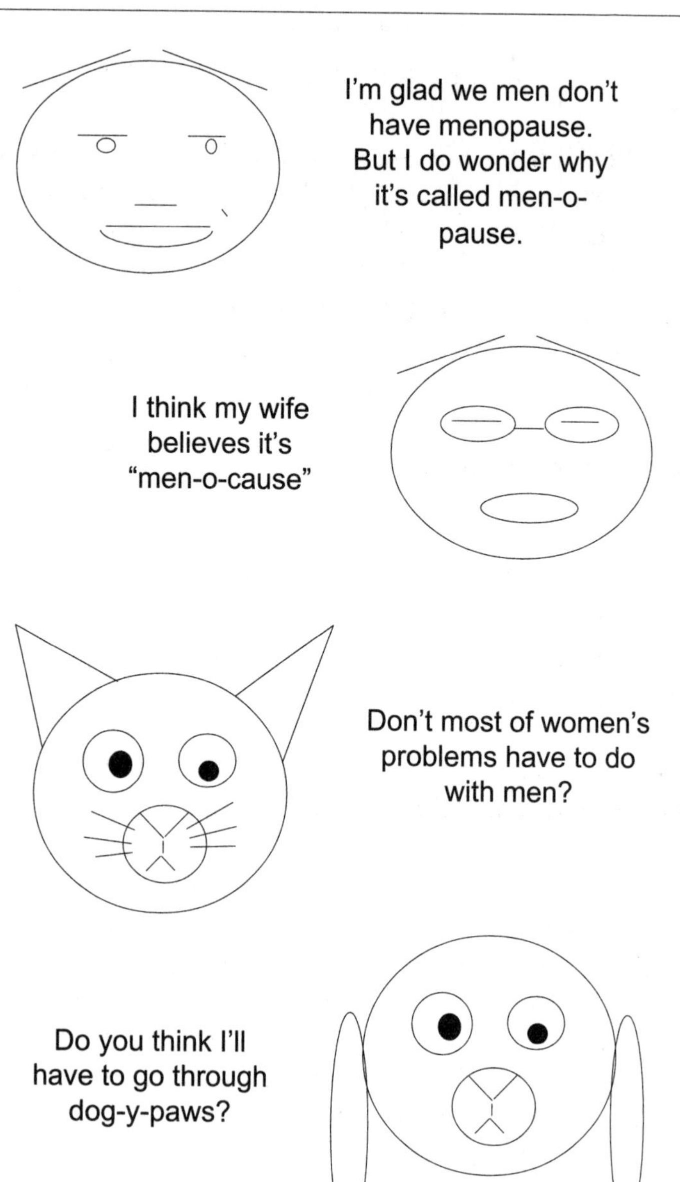
I'm glad we men don't have menopause. But I do wonder why it's called men-o-pause.
I think my wife believes it's "men-o-cause"
Don't most of women's problems have to do with men?
Do you think I'll have to go through dog-y-paws?

Chapter Five

Stress and the Stress Response

Why is there a decline of hormone levels? Is this decline natural? Not necessarily! There are causes for the decline and the chief of all is *stress.* Somewhat more complex than is insinuated by this well-worn-word, hormonal decline also results from an unskilled or dysfunctional response to stress. Much more significant is the question on how the stress got there in the first place. Yet let's postpone this question. *The biggest factors that cause reduction of hormone levels are imbedded in the creation of stress and having a dysfunctional response to it!*

In the 1950's Dr. Hans Selye, a physician from Montreal, wrote a book called The Stress of Life, which was a culmination of his research on stress. He shed light on the question of diminished hormones when he detailed the biological effects and consequences of the "stress response." This is the same stress response which I referred to earlier, where stress provokes a mobilization of our hormones.

His research showed that in the mobilization for "fight or flight" many physiological events take place. Think of the example of an attack by a saber-toothed tiger. He pointed out that under these circumstances, a biological response is launched in us that renders us ferocious enough to fight or flee. At the forefront of this mobilization is the massive outpouring of our adrenal stress hormones. These adrenal hormones raise the rate, power, and efficiency of the heart. They also strengthen our muscles, raise blood glucose to provide more fuel, and increase emotional fervor giving us strength to do what we need to do. As this happens, other systems are down regulated. Intestine, immune, reproduction, and other systems must donate their energy and resources to the common critical cause of survival.

Dr. Selye pointed out that when we are chronically stressed over time, the systems of our entire body will rise to the occasion and compensate. Our glands will enlarge and "rev up" production to keep up with the demands for greater quantities of stress hormones. For example, our thyroid gland will increase its production of thyroid hormones both to increase metabolism and to assist the adrenal gland.

The problem is that over time, the body is unable to sustain function at this heightened level. We cannot continue producing hormones at such an accelerated pace to cope with the high stress. Our glands begin to fatigue, decompensate, and hormone production diminishes. It is this attrition, from the long-term adaptation to stress, that we are observing in the hormone decline charts in figures 5, 6 and 7.

Since stress is the principle diminisher of the hormonal system, the question "is menopause as we know it, entirely natural" becomes strikingly pertinent. If we were not so stressed, would the decline in ovarian and other hormones be so serious? Could cycling and menstruation continue on for years or decades longer? Would we 'age' in the same way?

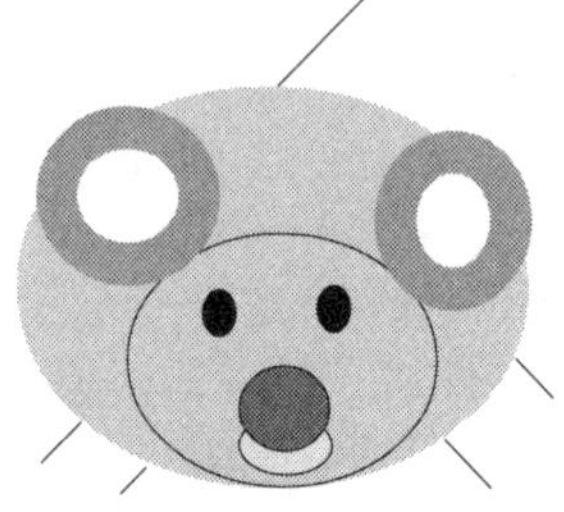

Wow! Yikes. Really?

It is not hard to imagine that it is natural and beneficial for women to cease ovulating, menstruating and having babies at a reasonable time in their life, and that this is built into the genetic programming. It may be that the origin of the *problems* of menopause can be caused from excessive hormonal decline from stress. We also need to consider that there are many women who have had little or no problems with menopause. It is the excessive hormonal diminishing originating from stress that can make menopause an unpleasant or even unhealthy experience.

So much that we have considered to be 'aging' is now felt to be the direct result of many causes that diminish our hormonal and other systems. Most of these causes boil down to compromised nutrition, toxicity and stress. Some refer to this decline as 'senescence' rather than 'aging.' We do not actually know what 'natural aging' looks like because, throughout history, we have been living out high levels of ongoing stress. So what would menopause and life be like if we were not so stressed?

We do not actually know what 'natural aging' looks like

Not stressed?! Is this possible? Perhaps a more relevant question would be "is stress natural?" All of us have stress in our lives. The stress did not die out after the era of saber-toothed tigers. Difficult events in our lives today cause an

Perhaps a more relevant question would be "is stress natural?"

identical physiologic response to that of the tiger challenge. There are the obvious stresses that appear to originate from issues of 'cash flow,' relationships, sex, illness, and global politics, to name a few. However these stresses pale in comparison to our failure to identify and fulfill our deepest dreams. These dreams are often ignored out of our forgetting and even denying what we really desire, need and want.

Often ignored stress results in forgetting and even denying what we really desire, need and want

Even as we begin exploring our dreams, we don't often really believe that we can have fulfillment of them. Because of this we may give up on our dreams and our deeper and more real ambitions. We may lack courage to continue dreaming and choosing what really matters to us. The stresses resulting from not living up to our destiny and dreams of love, happiness, fun, success, and spirituality are the most significant stresses of all.

High quality information, tools and support are now available to assist in the understanding and healing of stress in your life. Much of the stress of daily life is fueled from unresolved emotions and beliefs from the past that have been repressed away from conscious recognition and feel-

The most significant stresses result from not living up to our destiny and dreams of love, happiness, fun, success, and spirituality

ing. Guidance and tools are available to unveil and heal held fear, sadness, anger, shame and guilt as well as the distortions to thinking and believing that so interfere with perceiving, choosing and creating a great life. You can acquire these tools and be the principle guide to yourself in a healing process. You can also receive support from like-minded and skilled friends as well as talented and dedicated professionals.

Extra added stress can come from the way in which we respond (or do not respond) to the stress that we create. It is possible (and even quite common) to respond to stress in a dysfunctional or non-creative way and produce even more stress. This additional stress can worsen any situation by several magnitudes of difficulty and pain, and exaggerate the biological stress response!

Any current event in your life that is not beneficial will generate uncomfortable feelings. Clear and sometimes strong feelings are natural and they are part of our feedback mechanism that informs us that something is distinctly not okay. These feelings are quite intense at times, and correctly so, especially if there is something not quite right. If for example, issues regarding relationship, and communication are not listened to, honored, or responded to, ill feelings can be compounded.

Uncomfortable events can also trigger feelings that have been held in your 'emotional body.' For example, it is possible for couples to carry hidden resentment and burst out in anger at one another. At times the intensity of the outburst is excessive and just not in proportion or appropriate to the current difficulty.

An excessive response can have ancient origins. For example, a woman may not have been recognized, loved or adored by her father when she was a girl, and may carry forward an expectation that her husband will never love her enough and will disappoint her. This can color day to day interaction with her husband, and lead to greater disappointment and upset than a minor incident of neglect would ordinarily evoke.

For another example, a man that felt chronically unloved by his mother when he was a boy might have a chip on his shoulder. He might harbor a hidden resentment that his wife never loves him enough or in the right way. Therefore he may have hidden hostility and expectation resulting from unresolved anger that he has not healed from his past. He may add extra verbal punch to any tense situation. A current event can trigger the outpouring of past emotions: current pain can be amplified considerably by unresolved emotions, lingering from the past, slipping through.

Hidden resentment can result in one partner withholding love or authentic expression of their feelings toward the other. This diminishes intimacy, and creates a gap between the couple's connection. Over time, more and more distance can result and this process can be very destructive for the relationship. In this situation, intense feelings are often held in and denied, and expressed indirectly in ways that hurt the other partner. These feelings, when they are repressed, can also be translated into outbursts targeted to attack the other. Attacks can damage the relationship. Trust diminishes. Attraction deteriorates.

Leaking through of unhealed past emotions into a current situation can be an important factor in the origin of a dysfunctional response to current stress. Unfinished, unhealed emotions, coupled with the unbeneficial beliefs associated with them, distort perception of current situations and often lead to faulty, unbeneficial choices. At times the poor choices are not so significant and merely put a ruffle in our day. At other times the poor choices are profound, and can result for example, in lifelong marriages that are unbeneficial, or business partnerships that are destructive.

Emotional healing is the first step in developing a functional approach to dealing with and reducing stress. Emotional healing begins with recognizing, honoring and feeling your emotions. This does not mean that you leak out your emotions onto others. It means that you feel your emotions and that you are responsible for healing yourself. Choosing to be open, honest, accepting, compassionate and loving with yourself is essential. Making the right choices to heal and to be responsible, to provide a safe place for love, will lead you to the well-being that you desire.

Choice is the key. It is important to make 'right' choice the best that you can. 'Right' choice does not mean that you have made a perfect choice. That would be personal blackmail. 'Right' choice means that you make a choice that adds more complexity and authenticity to your life. Does the choice you make lead you to becoming a more honest, loving person to yourself and then to your partner? Does your choice help you know more about who you really are? Does it enhance your life and the life of your partner?

Making 'right' choice can help you create a life with

less stress, because each choice will result in your receiving more of the kind of life that reflects more of who you really are, and of what you really want.

Choice is the key.
Right choice,
wise choice,
empowered choice,
sacred choice.

Making 'wise' choices is also necessary. These choices are made by seeing the bigger picture, as well as the current one. Wise choices are choices made by using logic and reason, then letting that go and moving beyond logic and reason, so that you can allow your intuition and inner knowing to guide you.

Through making more right and wise choices in your life, a more positive future of dreams can be chosen, no matter what past issues that you or your partner have created for yourselves. You can begin new again. With responsibility (being willing to respond in a way that reflects the best of who you can be), you can catapult yourself into a life where you more elegantly create and express what really matters to you. As you do this, you give your body a break from the stress, and your body automatically heals itself. Your body is just waiting for you to take that *pause* that it needs so that it can do the healing it knows how to do!

There is far more to the healing process than I am describing here. If you want to know more about it, seek out the information, tools, and support. You will find it. With intention, mystically, "it will find you." With powerful individual healing there will be global healing. I believe it is possible to have a future without stress and without deterioration from the stress of unfulfilled dreams of love and life.

A future is possible without stress and without the deterioration from the stress of unfulfilled dreams of love and life

In summary, I propose that hormonal decline is, not 'natural.' Again, it is my belief that this form of decline is due to the effects of stress, both emotional and physiological, on our bodies.

I propose that hormonal decline is not 'natural'

There is an interesting illustration about how our view of aging can be challenged, and to support a possible contrast to senescence. Deep in the mountains of Mexico dwells a tribe of Indians known for their long distance runners. Interestingly, runners of this tribe reach peak performance at the age of sixty. Twenty year olds, within this culture run slower than sixty year

Hormonal decline is due to the effects of stress and a dysfunctional response to it, on our bodies

olds. Although it is not the sole reason for this achievement, these runners could not have performed this way at age sixty had their hormone levels significantly decreased. People within this culture did not consider it a natural process to have a loss of vitality and strength over time.

I raise the question, given proper care, great living, and exemplary treatment of our bodies, does our hormonal system need to decline?

Given proper care, great living, and, exemplary treatment of our bodies, does our hormonal system need to decline?

Chapter Six

Understanding Your Personal Hormone Needs

Hormonal Balance

Now let's advance further towards the treatment of menopause. As we have discussed, treating menopause with precision requires an understanding of hormonal balance and variation, as well as individual diversity and biological differences. Though as human beings we share a lot in common biologically, we also have many differences. Dr. Roger Williams researched and wrote about biological individuality. He pointed out that there are large variations in individual nutritional needs. For example, some people may do well with a certain 'RDA' or "Recommended Daily Allowance" of Vitamin B3, but others may need a few hundred times that dose to function normally.

There are large variations in individual needs

A Canadian Psychiatrist, Dr. Abram Hoffer brought this principle of biological individuality into his practice. He treated schizophrenics in a Saskatchewan mental institution with very large doses of vitamins (termed "megadose"), and was able to discharge many patients that resumed normal functioning on these high doses. One patient of his went on to become a prominent Canadian Psychiatrist! Dr. Hoffer was able to bring many people to health through administration of megadose vitamins.

Before treating people with medicines, herbs, hormones,

or vitamins, it is imperative we understand and respect the biological and biochemical individuality and sensitivity of each person. This is true in every aspect of medicine. Some patients are quite sensitive and will respond to a small dose of a medicine. Whereas others require a larger dose to elicit an adequate response. The variation in dosage from one individual person to another can be dramatic.

This is very relevant in treating women in menopause with hormones. Some need a tiny bit. Some need quite a bit. Some absorb well. Some absorb poorly. Some seem to need a hormone yet do poorly on any dose. Here we have other reasons to individualize.

Before treating people with medicines, herbs, hormones, or vitamins, it is imperative we understand and respect the biological and biochemical individuality of each person.

Besides the intricacies of biochemical individuality and the differences in sensitivities involved, women display differences in their internal balance of ovarian hormones. Each woman differs in the relative amount of her own estrogens, progesterone and testosterone levels. Body types give us indications of these variations in hormone levels and balance in women. There are infinite differences in body types possible. Hormones can play a role in this. For example, estrogens accelerate the closure of long bones and stimulate breast development. A woman who has higher estrogen levels early in life, will tend to be of shorter stature with larger breasts. A taller, smaller-breasted woman may have lower levels of estrogens earlier in life. There are many exceptions to these general descriptions of course, because there are many other determinants of body shape and size. There are many other symptoms, physical signs and laboratory markers that point to what your hormone levels were and are. Information on your personal hormone variances, throughout your life, will help in the design of your menopausal hormone strategy. Often a program that follows a hormone balance similar to what you have been accustomed to earlier in life, feels and works best.

A graphic representation, in figures 8 that follow, show three different estrogen patterns.

The first, figure 8a below, represents the hormonal configuration of a woman who has a balance in her estrogens, progesterone and testosterone levels.

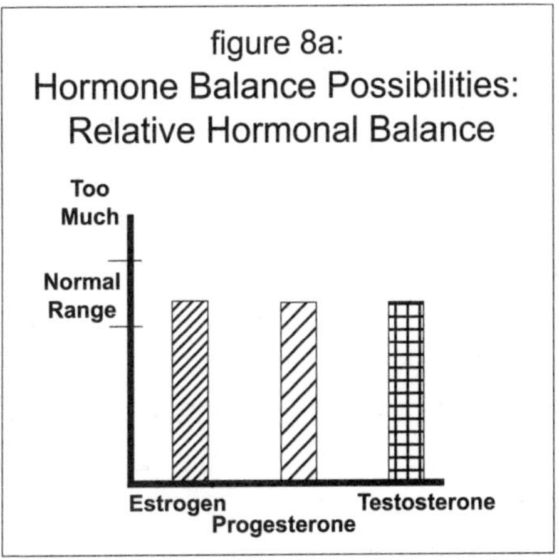

A second graph, in figure 8b below, represents a woman with a relatively large amount of estrogen.

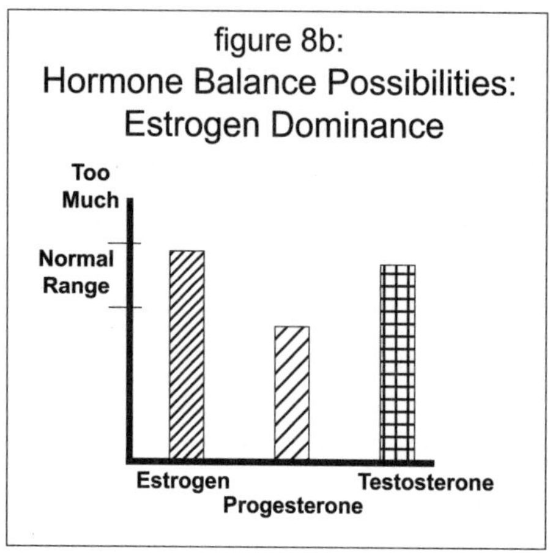

In a third graph, in figure 8c below, we see a relatively low amount of estrogen.

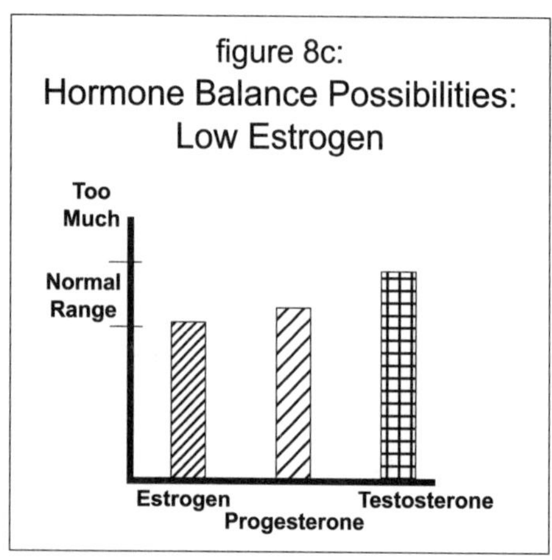

You can imagine the number of variables and variations that we can be dealing with clinically, especially as we include variations in the amounts of progesterone and testosterone as well.

So, you can see from these three different patterns for example, that a woman who had relatively lower amounts of estrogen all of her menstrual life should not need a large amount of estrogen during menopause. Her body would not be used to that and would not do well with it. On the other hand, a woman who has been used to generous amounts of estrogen, and had an abrupt fall of estrogen levels at menopause, will need adequate amounts of estrogens to feel good.

Women display differences in their unique and personal balance of ovarian hormones

Estrogen Dominance

A common circumstance that results in estrogen dominance exists when there is no ovulation, as depicted in figure 4 on page 19 and in figure 9 below. Earlier we touched on the fact that if ovulation does not occur, there is no significant progesterone production.

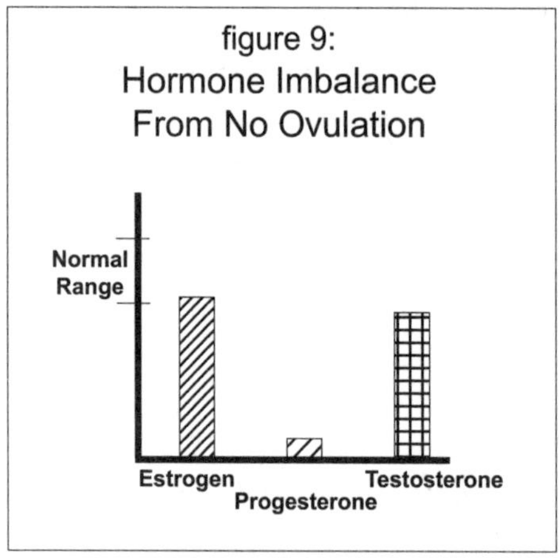

Lack of ovulation can occur at different times throughout a woman's life. Commonly, young women do not ovulate, or ovulate irregularly during the years of the onset of menstruation known as 'menarche'. Even though ovaries begin secreting estrogens in early adolescence, the secretion of estrogen does not depend upon ovulation. These secreted estrogens stimulate the development of breasts and uterine lining, and menstruation can occur even before ovulation begins. These 'anovulatory' periods, periods where there is no ovulation, can be very painful because the balancing and 'quieting' effects of progesterone are not in place to counteract the stimulation of estrogens. Recall that ovulation is required to produce adequate progesterone.

Failure to ovulate can occur again during

perimenopause, the time in your life just prior to the cessation of menstruation: ovulation can become erratic or cease entirely. Thus, in perimenopause when there is no ovulation, estrogen dominance is occurring. Once again, the stimulatory effects of estrogens are present without the balance of progesterone. Women may experience very difficult bouts of PMS, cramps, breast tenderness, and more, under these circumstances.

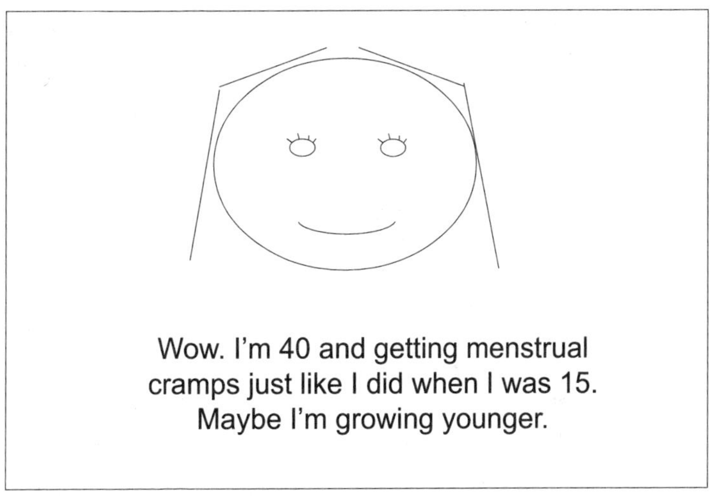

This significant abnormal phenomenon of anovulatory cycles that can occur prior to menopause is so much more prevalent than ever before. Four decades ago the average age of cessation of menstruation coincided with the average age of cessation of ovulation, which was forty-five years old. Today, in the western world, the average age of cessation of menstruation is anywhere from 45 - 51, while the average age of cessation of ovulation is 10 years earlier: 35! Therefore there can be up to a decade, or even more of excessive stimulation by estrogens not balanced by progesterone!

I believe that this drastic change in cessation of ovulation by a factor of ten years has several causes. One serious contributor is that estrogens are injected into and sprayed onto our food supply. Direct administration of these hormones to dairy cattle and beef, as well as indirect consumption through estrogen active toxic herbicides and pesticides in the animal feed, are standard procedure on cattle ranches. For many decades estrogens have been injected into cattle to fatten them for market and to increase milk production.

After World War II there was a major surplus of ammunition nitrates. These were put to use as fertilizers to enhance plant growth. Nitrates were placed on the soil and the plants did grow. However because these fertilizers lacked other essential elements, such as minerals, necessary for plant health, unhealthy plants developed. These plants became more vulnerable to insects and fungi. The response to this new problem was the production and widespread use of herbicides and pesticides. These substances unfortunately happen to have estrogen-like effect on the human body!

The introduction of these estrogenic effectors into the food supply has been sufficient enough, and is the probable cause behind the change of the average age of the onset of menses, menarche, from 13 to 11. Today it is not uncommon to see 9 year old girls with initial breast development. Visible signs of hormonal imbalance are surfacing as early as nine years into the development of a child! These premature changes can be directly attributed to the food entering your child's mouth. The disarming prevalence of hormonal imbalances and related illness speaks deeply of the need to have quality knowledge about health and your body...and to revamp the food supply!

Not only are these chemicals estrogenic, they are toxic. After all, it takes strong poisons to kill these durable insects and fungi on plants. The hormones that are injected into animals, and the agricultural chemical herbicides and pesticides are fat-soluble. When the pesticides deposit in the fat in breast tissue, you have toxic and stimulating substances in close proximity to vulnerable, changeable, breast glandular tissue. This contact between poisonous chemicals and vulnerable breast tissue makes the breast tissue more susceptible to cancer. When these poisons deposit in the fat tissue in the waistline, where there are mostly fat cells, which do not readily change, the vulnerability to cancer there, is much less.

Increasing estrogen dominance is one of the causes of the astronomical rise in occurrence of breast, uterine and ovarian disease. Over-stimulation of the uterine lining by estrogen and estrogenic-like compounds can also lead to endometriosis and even endometrial cancer. Over-stimulation of the breast glandular tissue can lead to enlargement of the breasts, fibrocystic disease, and worse. In addition,

Increasing estrogen dominance is one of the causes of the astronomical rise in breast, uterine and ovarian disease

over-stimulation of the muscular uterine wall by estrogen can lead to fibroid tumors. Fibroids, in turn, can lead to excessive uterine bleeding that results in countless hysterectomies. Because estrogen production is diminished during menopause, one cure for fibroids may be menopause. Better still, many hysterectomies that have occurred before menopause could have been, *and can be*, averted by early detection and treatment of the progesterone deficiency, which has resulted from premature cessation of ovulation, and ensuing estrogen dominance.

One of my patients, at the age of 35, was diagnosed with a uterine fibroid the size of a large navel orange. She was told it had to be surgically removed. She went to the library to read about fibroids and discovered, in her words, that they "feed on estrogen." At that time many of her friends, who were runners, had stopped having their periods (probably because the stress of excessive running diverted resources destined to become ovarian hormones to other needed adrenal hormones). She believed that periods were caused by estrogens and therefore if she ran hard enough and long enough she could stop her periods. She believed that this would "stop the estrogen," and thus, again in her words, "starve the fibroid." She ran for 3 miles a day for 3 months until her period stopped, and then for another month until the "fibroid starved" and disappeared. I mention this to illustrate a point regarding excessive estrogens, not necessarily to endorse her method (though not too shabby an approach!)

Many hysterectomies before menopause can be averted by early detection and treatment of progesterone deficiency.

Estrogen dominance can also originate from other

causes. Thirty years ago, when a young woman showed up in a doctor's office with PMS and breast tenderness she was probably not ovulating. Therefore, she was not producing progesterone and had symptoms from unopposed estrogen. Today when a young woman complains of these uncomfortable symptoms, there is just as strong a probability that her liver is not adequately breaking down the estrogens that she is producing and as a result, estrogens accumulate and become excessive.

The liver, which has so many crucial functions in our body, runs into many problems today. Difficulties primarily result from toxins in the food, pollutants in the environment, alcohol, pharmaceutical and street drugs, as well as toxic consequences from under-discovered infection in the intestines. All of these are present in great excess in our times, and continually bombard the liver detoxification system.

Your body's management of estrogen throughout the menstrual cycle is complex. Estrogens that are produced are processed biochemically, conjugated, and excreted by the liver. Optimal estrogen hormone levels are maintained in this way. However, estrogens are often not broken down properly by the liver. Excessive detoxification chores from external and internally generated toxins impair liver function. Externally acquired toxins can eventually overload a liver. Toxins produced internally by intestinal infection flow through the lymph system to the liver, and eventually can play a role in impairing estrogen processing. Both situations will affect the liver and cause estrogen dominance. We can often treat menstrual and menopausal symptoms by helping the liver. Also, when there is difficulty in the liver, we have an increased possibility that aggressive unsafe estrogen metabolites will result. We will discuss this later.

The birth control pill is another serious factor that contributes to excessive estrogen stimulation. "The pill" contains hormones that have a different molecular structure than natural ovarian hormones. Because of the artificial part of the molecules, they will behave somewhat differently in the body than real hormones, and they will require additional liver processing. Birth control pills contain only aggressive altered estrogens with no balance from *natural* progesterone. It violates common sense and safety to give additional hormones to young women, who already have an abundance of hormones. Over the years, the medical field has had experience with the administration of excessive amounts of hormones. It always results in problematic "side effects."

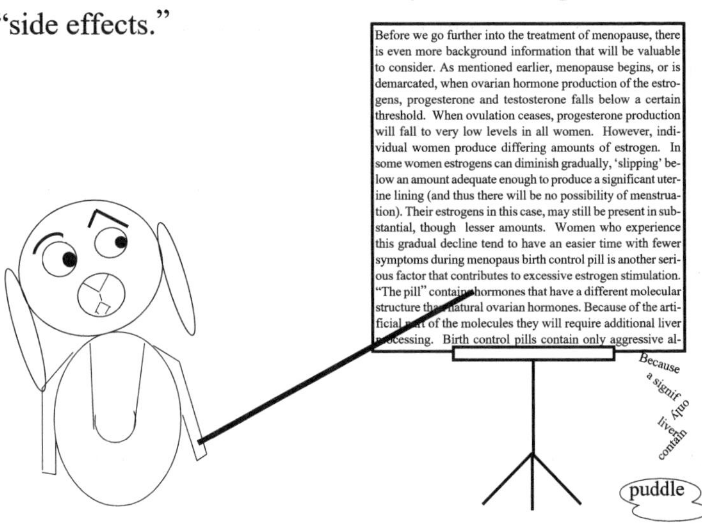

Chapter Seven

Further Background On Menopause

We have more background information that will be valuable to consider. As mentioned earlier, menopause begins, or is demarcated, when ovarian hormone production falls below a certain threshold. When ovulation ceases, progesterone production will fall to very low levels in all women.

However, individual women produce differing amounts of the estrogens. In some women estrogens can diminish gradually, 'slipping' below an amount adequate enough to produce a significant uterine lining (and thus there will be no possibility of menstruation). Their estrogens in this case, may still be present in substantial, though lesser amounts. Women who experience this gradual decline tend to have an easier time with fewer symptoms during menopause. This situation is depicted in figure 10a below.

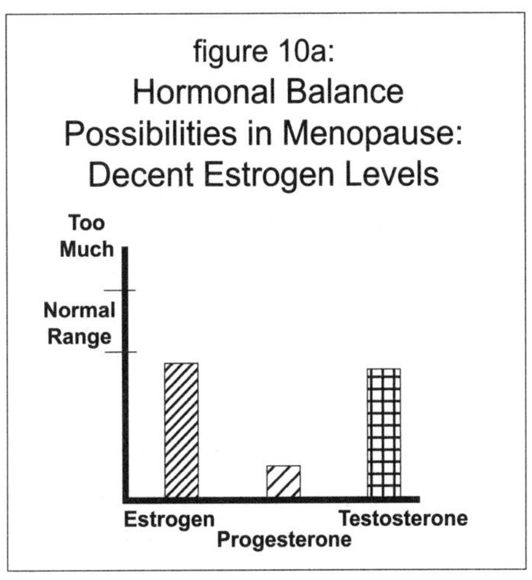

At the other extreme, seen in figure 10b below, there can be a precipitous decline in estrogen amounts. Women who experience this type of estrogen loss will often have many symptoms and a more difficult time. Many possible variations in rate and level of estrogen decline exist within these two extremes.

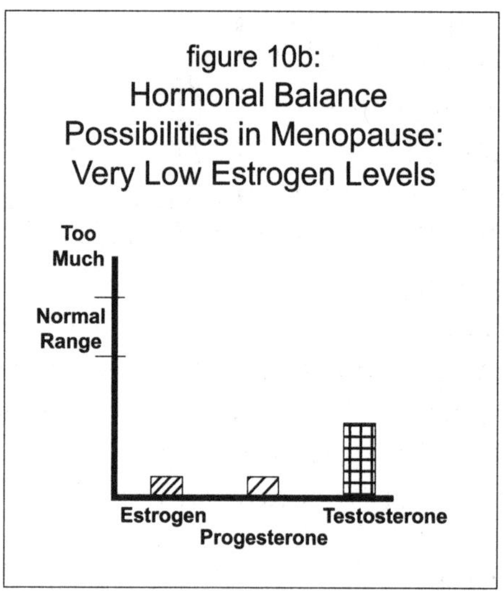

figure 10b:
Hormonal Balance
Possibilities in Menopause:
Very Low Estrogen Levels

It is also common to find oscillating and surging levels of estrogens during menopause. Oscillating and surging are accompanied by symptoms like 'hot flashes' and night sweats. Proper treatment, as well as living in comfort during this transitional time in your life, may require identifying individual differences in hormonal needs.

We have learned from some misconceptions and mistakes of the past. For example, in the past problems developed when the 'one-dose-fits-most' prescriptions of estrogens, with no progesterone to balance, were given. This type of dosing could work somewhat well for a woman who entered menopause with very low estrogen levels. The additional estrogen would elevate her into decent hormone levels, as you can see in figure 11a to the right. However, each woman is different, and therefore, enters into menopause with different estrogen levels. A woman whose estrogen levels remain substantial (as illustrated in figure 11b below) yet have slipped below amounts sufficient to menstruate, will do best with a more subtle dose. When she is given the common 'one-size-fits-most' dose of estrogen, she will wind up with excessive amounts of total estrogen. This is unacceptable and can be dangerous.

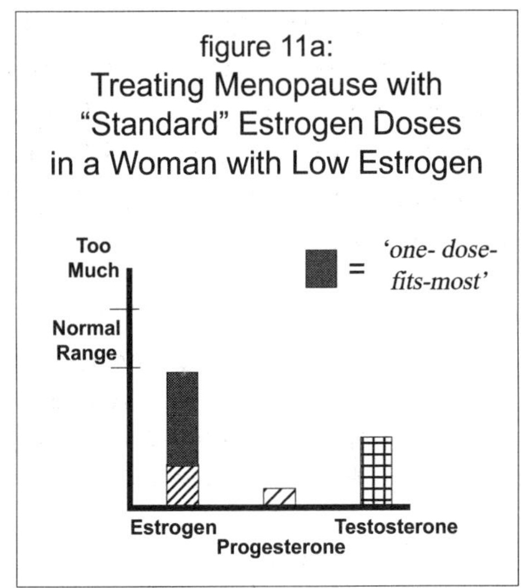

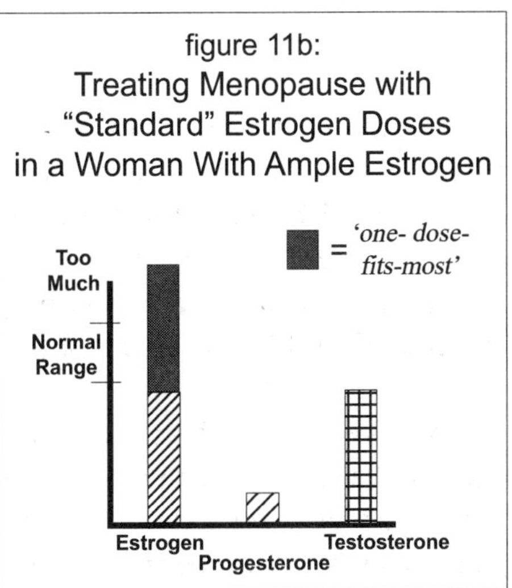

A primary goal of the treatment of

menopause is to find *accurate* doses of hormones for treatment of each *individual* woman, as shown in the figures below. In figure 12a, the woman who has very low estrogen levels is given substantial doses of estrogen. In figure 12b, the woman with very substantial estrogen is given very low doses, if any. Failure to adequately recognize and address these significant differences in hormonal balance in individual women is a problem. Earlier I mentioned that there have been, and are, less-than-optimal treatment approaches to menopause: 'one-dose-fits- most' is one of the most prevalent.

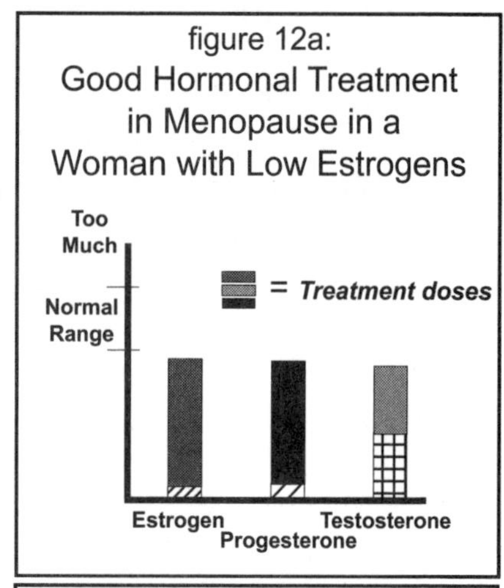

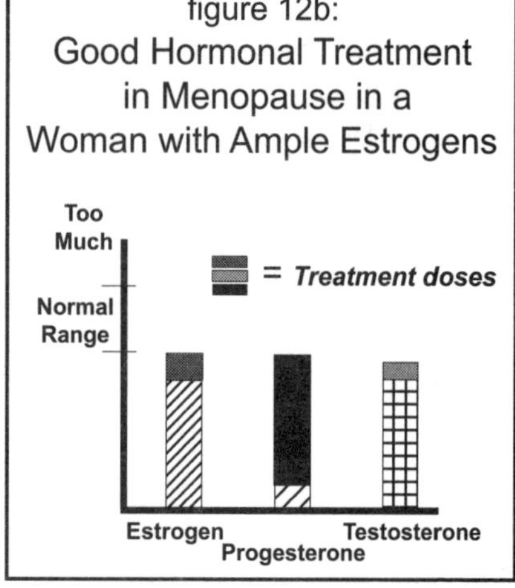

The second example of an outdated conception, is the belief that progesterone was not relevant at menopause. The theory was that since there was no anticipation of pregnancy there was no need for treatment with progesterone. Therefore, it was thought that progesterone was relevant only for cycling and pregnancy. However, women who are treated with estrogens alone do not have the balancing and protective benefit of progesterone, and we now know where that can lead... discomfort and harm to your health!

A Common Menopause Occurrence

The most common situation encountered in women who are approaching, or have entered early menopause, is that of reduced or negligible amounts of progesterone. Once again, a precipitous loss of progesterone occurs when ovulation ceases. Also, as we have emphasized, this will be coupled with a variable reduction, individual to individual, in estrogen levels. When ovulation ceases there is negligible and insufficient progesterone to balance estrogens. This occurs along with an overall reduction of estrogen levels, which is also taking place in perimenopause.

In the midst of all this talk of progesterone deficiency, it is important to remember that estrogen can be necessary as well. When estrogen levels fall below a threshold, significant or serious symptoms can arise. Even in this circumstance of reduced estrogens, estrogen *dominance* may still occur, and the symptoms of it may be experienced. Estrogen, when in diminished amounts, still needs to be accompanied by ample progesterone to maintain balance.

It is also important to realize that minimal to severe reductions in testosterone levels, again varying woman to woman, can be occurring as well.

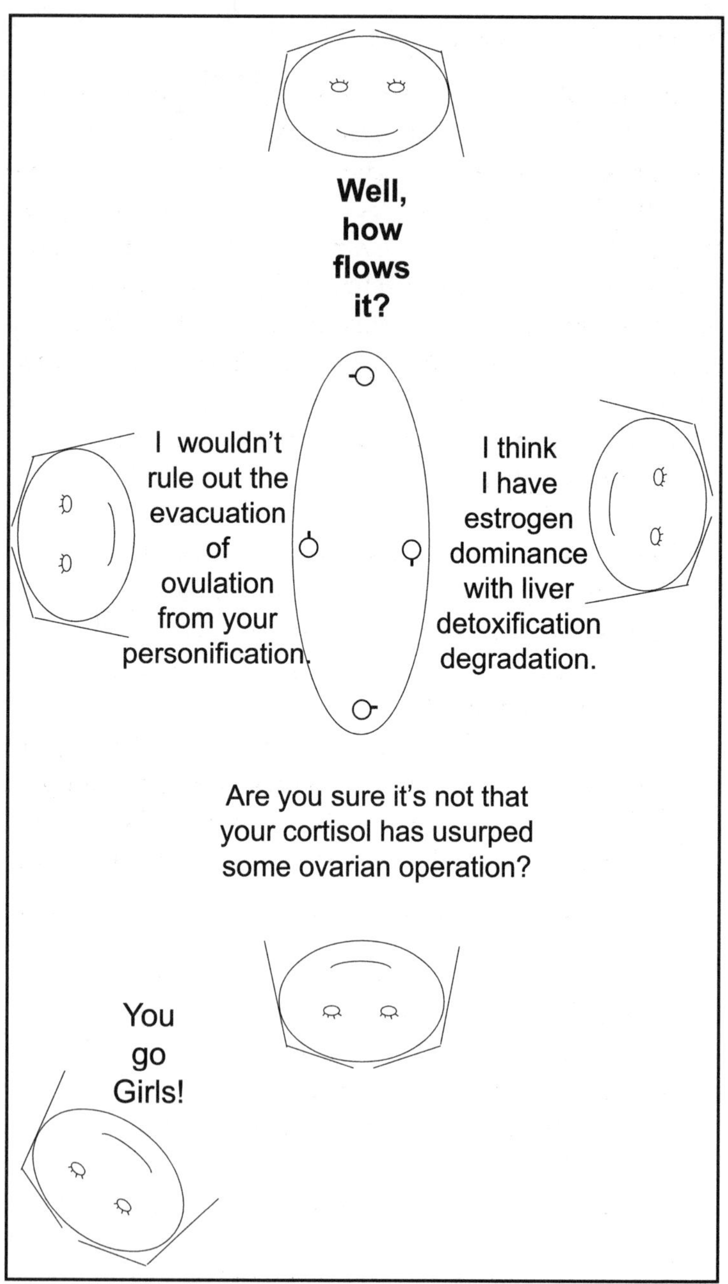
Well, how flows it?
I wouldn't rule out the evacuation of ovulation from your personification.
I think I have estrogen dominance with liver detoxification degradation.
Are you sure it's not that your cortisol has usurped some ovarian operation?
You go Girls!

A Hormonal Questionnaire

In my practice, in order to learn more about each individual woman, we acquire information from a hormonal questionnaire, as seen in figures 13a, b & c on pages 63 through 65. This information can help us characterize your profile of hormone levels, hormone balance and risk factors for illness. This can also help us have more clarity and specificity in treatment. I'd like to add that this technique has been taken to an art through the work of a Naturopathic physician, Dr. Joseph Collins, on Menopausal Type. For those interested in this useful approach, refer to the website *www.yourmenopausetype.com* or Dr. Collins' book.

The answers to the questions on menarche on our questionnaire hint at a woman's hormonal undertone. They suggest intensity of hormonal output, unveil initial imbalances, and reveal greater relative proportions of estrogen, progesterone or testosterone. Birth control methods, pregnancy and lactation information all add to the understanding of risk factors. PMS and breast tenderness, signs of estrogen dominance recurring after age 35, help clue us in to a possible early cessation of ovulation, and thus an early need

Our questionnaire is useful to get a general idea about:

* your hormonal balance between estogens, progesterone and testosterone early in life;
* suggestions of whether or not you are currently deficient in estrogens, progesterone and/or testosterone;
* your specific risk factors for female organ illness and osteoporosis.

for progesterone. Information about women who feel best only at mid-cycle or during pregnancy tells us they are probably marginal in their estrogen levels and enjoy the higher levels of estrogen present at these times. Breast feeding and bra wearing time gives additional information regarding cancer risk. Breast size and tenderness reflect estrogen levels or lack of progesterone balance.

The questions in figure 13b on mid-page 64 again address risk factors. Height, weight, and increase in breast size all reflect different types of estrogen prevalence or dominance, and give clues regarding osteoporosis (if there is loss of height). Specific symptoms of estrogen, progesterone and testosterone deficiencies lead to understanding the specific needs for these hormones.

The questions in figure 13c focus you directly to possible symptoms from hormone inadequacy or imbalance.

figure 13a: Hormone Questionnaire page 1

Current Age_________
Approximate date of last menstrual period _________
Approximate date of last menstrual period
at time when your periods were regular_________
Age of onset of menstruation (Menarche) _________
How long after Menarche did your periods get regular?____months
How many days did your menstrual flow last? _______
What was cycle length when periods got regular?
(from one first day of cycle to the next) _______

Prior to the age of 18 or, your first pregnancy:
did you have "PMS" ___yes __no
did you have difficult periods ___yes __no
breast tenderness ___yes __no
headaches ___yes __no irritablility: ___yes __no
uterine cramps ___yes __no heavy flow ___yes __no

birth control methods: __Diaphragm __Condom __both
__IUD [__# of years] __tubal ligation
Were you ever on the Birth Control Pill? ___yes __no
__# of years or __# of months
If 'yes', how did you feel on it? ___better ___worse

Have you ever been pregnant & given birth? __no __yes
if yes, # of births ___
Your age at each pregnancy _____ _____ _____
Number of months you breast fed this baby _____ _____ _____
After the first 3 months was pregnancy
a very physically pleasant time for you? ___yes __no
a worse time for you than non-pregnant? ___yes __no
Number of ___miscarriages ___abortions

Have you had a recurrance or worsening
premenstrual symptoms after the age of 35? ___yes ___no
After the age of 35, before menopause,
Is there a time of the month that you feel best?
week: __1 __2: __3: __4
Is this the only time of the month you feel good? ___yes __no

figure 13b: Hormone Questionnaire page 2

Breast size when younger or, prior to first pregnancy
__small __medium __large
Current breast size: __smaller than above __ larger

have you had any of the following breast problems?
__ cysts ___ biopsy ___ cancer __abnormal mammogram
have you had mammograms? ___no __yes: number___
any abnormalities (describe)____________________
do you have breast implants? ___yes ___no
if yes, for how many years ____
what percentage of time in a 24 hour day do you wear a bra? ___%

Have you had any of the following:

__uterine fibroids ___D & C [__# of] __ovarian cysts
__endometriosis __laparoscopic surgeries __cesarian sections
__hysterectomy __tubal ligation
__oopherectomy [removal of ovary(s)] __no __one __both
__abnormal pap smear
__Premarin __Provera __patch ___other hormones
[list]____________________

Has any woman in your family had female cancer? __no __yes
if yes, who and what type? __breast __uterine __ovarian
who? _______ _______ ________

Current Height ____feet ____inches
Tallest height you ever were____feet ____inches
Weight age 25____lbs Weight now ____lbs
In your life have you had more muscle and hair than others? ____
more muscle than others with little body hair? ____?

figure 13c: Hormone Questionnaire page 3

Symptoms of estrogen deficiency:

__hot flashes __temperature swings __night sweats
__vaginal dryness __ racing mind @ night __trouble falling asleep
__mental fogginess ___depression __intestinal bloating
__diminished sexuality & sensuality __heart palpitations
__weight gain ___back & joint pain __headaches & migraines

Symptoms of estrogen excess:

__ breast tenderness (especially central)
__ breast swelling or enlarging
__ water retention & swelling __pelvic cramps __nausea
__ impatient & snappy though with clear mind

Symptoms of progesterone deficiency:

__difficulty sleeping __anxiety & nervousness __water retention
__no period __infrequent period __shorter cycle
__frequent & heavy periods __spotting before period ___PMS
__cystic breasts __painful breasts __endometriosis __fibroids

Symptoms of testosterone deficiency:

__diminished sex drive __flabbiness __muscle weakness
__diminished energy & stamina __diminished sense of security
__diminished coordination & balance __indecisiveness
__diminished armpit, pubic & body hair __hair loss
__diminished love of your body image

Chapter Eight
The Hormones Themselves

Let's look more closely at the three ovarian hormones: estrogens, progesterone and testosterone. Learning about these three hormones will help us gain a more solid understanding of how we create and administer individualized treatment programs for women when we use hormones.

Estrogens

Estrogens are a group of hormones that help to biologically define aspects of the 'feminine.' Estrogens initiate many of the physical changes that occur from girlhood to womanhood. Many of the feelings of being feminine are biologically derived from estrogen. Uzzi Reiss M.D., a gynecologist, in his clearly written book on menopause, Natural Hormone Balance for Women, states it well: "Estrogen makes you feel sensual. It brings glow to the skin, moisture to the eyes, fullness to the breasts, and clarity to the mind. It keeps the vagina lubricated. It uplifts and stabilizes your mood. It influences your brain and your bones, and protects you against cardiovascular disease..."

Estrogens are a group of hormones that help to biologically define aspects of 'feminine'

Estrogen deficiency symptoms arise when estrogen production slips. Vagina, skin and eyes can become dry. Mental fogginess can develop. Mood can dwindle and one's sense of temperature can fluctuate. Other changes that commonly occur are listed in figure 14 below and include:

- hot flashes and night sweats
- back and joint pain
- episodes of rapid heartbeat and palpitations
- headaches and migraines
- difficulty falling asleep
- diminished sense of sexuality and sensuality
- pain on intercourse
- weight gain
- sense of abdominal bloating
- sense of normalcy only during second week of cycle

figure 14: Estrogens

Estrogen makes you feel sensual. It brings glow to the skin, moisture to the eyes, fullness to the breasts, and clarity to the mind. It keeps the vagina lubricated. It uplifts and stabilizes your mood. It influences your brain and your bones, and protects you against cardiovascular disease..."

Uzzi Reiss M.D. Natural Hormone Balance for Women

Estrogen Deficiency

Dry vagina, eyes, and skin with loss of glow	Pain on intercourse
Temperature swings	Hot flashes and night sweats
Sleep Disturbance	Headaches and migraines
Back and joint pain	Fatigue and reduced stamina

Episodes of rapid heartbeat and palpitations
Mental fogginess and forgetfulness
Diminished sense of sensuality and sexuality
Weight gain, especially thighs, hips and buttox
Sense of intestinal bloating
Sense of normalcy only during second week of cycle

Estrogen Excess

Breast tenderness, especially central	Impatient but clear of mind
Water retention, swollen fingers & legs	Increase in breast size

Pelvic cramps, with or without bleeding

Progesterone

Progesterone has a variety of profound physiologic effects. It balances the effects of estrogen. It is calming to the nervous system. If it were to be injected intravenously it would cause a sleep deep enough for surgery to be performed. Also, progesterone is crucial in the deposition of bone, and facilitates the functioning of thyroid hormone. Adequate progesterone sustains pregnancy and the length of the menstrual cycle.

When progesterone is deficient we get a combination of adverse effects. Prior to menopause, when progesterone diminishes in amount, periods are affected. The actual onset of each menstruation is triggered by the natural fall in progesterone levels towards the end of each cycle. When progesterone production diminishes somewhat, spotting, or an earlier period can result. The word "progesterone" is derived from "pro-gestation" --supportive of pregnancy.

When ovulation fails to occur in any given menstrual cycle, far from sufficient progesterone is produced during that cycle. When ovulation ceases entirely, even though you may still have sufficient estrogen to build up (and shed) a uterine lining, progesterone diminishes dramatically. Finally, when ovulation and periods cease entirely, major progesterone deficiency is certain, and dramatic changes can occur.

Sleep disturbance can be a common and unwelcomed change. It can be mild, moderate or severe, and often results from the loss of the beneficial effect of progesterone. Another consequence of diminished progesterone on the brain can be mild, moderate or severe changes in mood and well-being. The effects of inadequate progesterone on sleep and mood can be profound.

Genna stands out in my memory regarding the power of progesterone. She is strong and quite successful in life. However, when I first saw her she wanted to impress upon me that even though she may look okay, she was absolutely falling apart! Every aspect of her life was in trouble and she felt miserable! After treating her with progesterone, within a reasonable amount of time she was happy, calm and had a huge smile! Progesterone can facilitate dramatic changes!

Progesterone augments thyroid hormone, which is crucial to vibrant metabolism and the burning of calories. Loss of progesterone is one of the several reasons that women can gain weight during menopause. Refer to figure 15 below for a list of progesterone deficiency symptoms.

figure 15: Progesterone Deficiency

Progesterone Deficiency

Sleep disturbance	Anxiety, depression & mood problems
Water Retention	Spotting a few days before period
Osteoporosis	No period, infrequent period
Sweet crave	Heavy and frequent periods
Delayed menarche	Difficulty getting pregnant
Weight Gain	Diminshing of Thyroid hormone effects

Progesterone Deficiency Leading to Estrogen Dominance

PMS	Fibroids, Endometriosis
Breast tenderness and pain	Breast lumps, cysts & +

There are other effects of lowered progesterone. These are more the result of the estrogen dominance which develops from the lack of progesterone balancing. These negative changes include breast tenderness, uterine fibroids, and endometriosis.

Testosterone

Testosterone energizes, rejuvenates, is essential for muscle and bone, supports mood and appropriate aggression, and is fundamental to female libido. Testosterone levels also diminish in menopause. The magnitude of the decrease will vary from woman to woman. Loss of libido is common. Many women who are accustomed to being strong in life can get unusually insecure or fearful as testosterone diminishes. Flab appearing under the arms can be from lower testosterone. Testosterone is an important part of treatment of some vaginal problems. Determining the need for testosterone, and supplementing it in menopausal women, can be very important!

Chapter Nine

Final Background to Treatment with Hormones

We are ready to ask a fundamental question of whether or not to treat menopause, and if the answer is "yes," what are the optimal ways to treat menopausal women? I believe it is often, but not always, beneficial to supplement hormones at menopause. In the context of so careful consideration of safety, elegant individualized treatment with hormones can make a wonderful difference in the present and the future.

We need to consider that millions of women have passed through menopause without receiving any hormonal or other treatment. Many women glide through it with ease, or without too much difficulty. Many others have moderate or even severe difficulties and feel very uncomfortable living inside their own skin. Even though all women have an overall loss of progesterone, the women who have adequate amounts of remaining estrogen, or who had lower estrogen levels earlier in life, may have an easier time going through menopause. Some women with apparent 'adequate' estrogens however, are exceptions and may also benefit from additional estrogens.

We also want to consider other factors that may lead to later difficulties in menopause from hormone deficiencies and imbalance. There are possible complications such as hip fractures from osteoporosis that are contributed to by hormone deficiency, for one example. Coronary artery disease, which may not show up until much later in life, is another example. There is debate about whether or not hormones are relevant to coronary problems in women. We know that there is some relationship, as the incidence of coronary problems is much less in premenopausal women, as compared to men of the same age. However, the ratio of this incidence in males and females equalizes after menopause.

When we consider whether or not to treat menopause, we return to the question: how 'natural' is menopause? I believe menopause, as we currently encounter or experience it, is significantly tempered and influenced by the general decline that takes place in all hormones in all women and men. Again, because special thresholds are involved, some symptoms are more dramatic. As I implied earlier, I believe overall hormonal decline is ultimately caused by a multitude of biological and emotional stress factors including difficult events occurring during our lives, emotional dysfunction, inadequacies of diet, toxins in our food and environment, untreated physiological deficiencies or diseases, hidden infections, and insufficient happiness, love, success and spirituality. This list could go on and on! Once again, evidence is strong that general hormonal decline, including decline of the ovarian hormones, is stress related.

I believe treatment is called for when uncomfortable symptoms appear, not only for the purpose of alleviating the discomfort, but also for the purpose of addressing the significant biological and emotional consequences of insufficient hormones. The spiraling effects of menopausal symptoms, such as hot flashes and sleep disturbance, can result in fatigue and irritability. Dwindling mood can cause significant deterioration in quality of life. Sexual dysfunction can lead to strained relationships. Bone mineral loss can be a setup for pain, debilitation and possible surgery.

This list of symptoms could continue further.

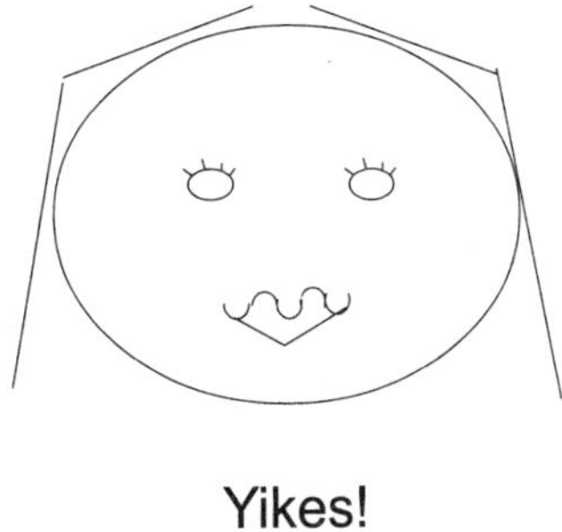

Yikes!

There have been claims and considerable evidence that treatment with hormones can also lead to difficulties, some severe. I suggest that these problems are largely due to inadequate risk assessment as well as faulty or not comprehensive enough treatment. You also must keep in mind, regarding hormones of any kind, that it is not healthy to have diminished levels of hormones. On the other hand, if hormonal supplementation results in exceeding normal hormone levels, known as 'overdose,' problems are guaranteed.

For example, taking excess doses of B vitamins will not result in any consequences outside of more expensive urine. However, overdose with hormones will sooner or later always cause a problem. Look what happened to millions of Americans put on cortisone circa the 1950's when it was first commercially available. Initially, many people felt very good. Their inflammatory symptoms as well as adrenal fatigue were relieved and they felt happier and less tired… that is before they ended up with serious side effects such as osteoporosis, immune suppression, muscle wasting and body fat redistribution. In the original exuberance to treat, overdose occurred. Excessive hormones lead to difficulties.

Another problem of treatment with ovarian hormones is that the vast majority of the hormones prescribed have been biologically different from human hormones. The artificial hormones are different molecularly from what ovaries produce. Initial mass production of estrogens began by capturing the urine of pregnant horses. Horses have similar, but by no means identical, estrogens to humans. A product called Premarin was produced. Pregnant mare urine was collected and the estrogens were isolated out.

The differences between horse and human estrogens themselves pose a major problem. Horses have an abundance of aggressive estrogens with none of the balancing estriol. They also contain estrogens peculiar to horses that are not present in humans, one of which is known to be toxic to genes. Animal-rights activists also point out that these horses have not been treated well. The mares are impregnated, placed in stalls, catheterized to collect all of their urine, and dehydrated to keep their urine concentrated. A pharmacist friend once asked me if I had ever noticed that the premarin pill had an especially thick coating. He said that he bit into it once, out of curiosity, and that the pill smelled strongly of horse urine! Scary!

As with so many situations in medicine, initial ideas have turned out to have unanticipated problems and side effects.

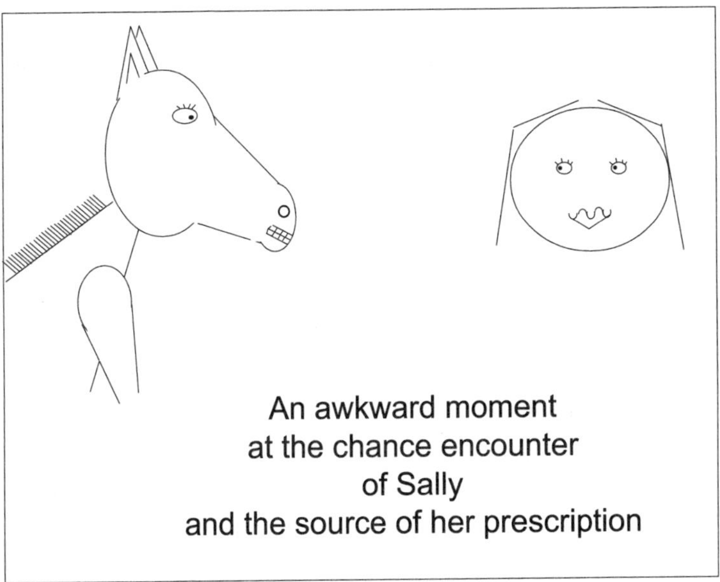

An awkward moment
at the chance encounter
of Sally
and the source of her prescription

Chapter Ten
Treatment With Hormones

Treatment with hormones requires evaluation and assessment of the needs and risk factors of each individual woman as well as consideration of the merits and risks of each of the three ovarian hormones.

Progesterone has many important functions, as I have demonstrated. So when ovulation ceases and progesterone declines, with few exceptions, it is hard for me to imagine a woman who would *not* benefit by taking progesterone. (An obvious exception would include women who had a breast cancer that had progesterone sensitive receptor sites. Though there is even controversy about this, in my opinion, treatment with progesterone in this case, would be contraindicated. There are other exceptions regarding treatment with progesterone, including women who for unknown reasons just do not do well on it).

It is crucial to consider estrogens with ample caution because of the adversities that occur from estrogen dominance. This is of course due to estrogen over-stimulation and its implications with regards to female organ illness. We consider it critical to take a close and careful look at possible risk factors such as the use of the birth control pill, estrogen levels earlier in life, number of pregnancies and lactations, family history, health history, and the technical processing of estrogens by your liver which is revealed by testing.

Testosterone treatment has its own intricacies. Biochemically, estrogens are produced from testosterone, as you can see in figure 2 on page 23. Therefore, any additional testosterone could add to the total amounts of estrogens. Also, excessive testosterone will have other symptoms all of its own, such as unwanted hair growth in unusual places.

Products Available

I want to point out, at this juncture, how important the type, quality, and source of hormones are to the outcome of the treatment of women. A lot has been learned and developed in the field of ovarian hormones. Three decades ago Jonathan Wright M.D. uncovered research from the 1960's regarding healthy ratios of the individual estrogens. This is the story of the beneficial influence of estriol that I mentioned earlier. Because of this discovery, pharmacists began to search for, and found, pure molecule-identical hormones from natural sources. From these sources they prepared, or "compounded," formulations that replicated exactly, human hormone biochemistry. Safe, bio-identical hormones were then made available for purchase.

Compounding pharmacists, ironically, purchase the pure hormones from pharmaceutical companies. These companies derive pure molecularly-identical hormones from soybeans. However, the pharmaceutical companies are not interested in these pure hormones as is. They cannot patent them because U.S. law prohibits the patenting of any molecule that exists in the human body. Instead, they alter these molecules in order to produce a 'patent medicine' from which they make a more substantial profit.

For example, the pharmaceutical companies extract pure

estradiol, alter it, and manufacture a substance called ethinyl estradiol. They take pure progesterone, alter it, and make 'norethindrone.' The problem with this alteration is that you introduce a molecule into the body that is different from one in the body. This altered "progestin" has more testosterone-like effects than it does progesterone-like effects. As norethindrone is a common constituent of birth control pills, consequences of this are widespread. Furthermore, the newly introduced foreign molecule has medicinal effects on the body that are different from a pure hormonal effect, and can produce what are called 'side effects.' Some of these side effects are harmful; others, though rare, can be lethal.

Fortunately today there are great molecularly-identical hormones derived from natural sources available to women! There are pharmacists in thousands of American and European cities and towns that compound these bio-identical hormones. You can find a compounding pharmacist in your area through the website of the International Academy of Compounding Pharmacists (IACP):

http://www.iacprx.org/about_iacp/

A compounding pharmacist is sure to know the doctors in your area who are knowledgeable and friendly to natural hormones.

Methods of Administration of Hormones

There are three common methods of administering ovarian hormones: transdermal preparations, oral capsules, and sublingual drops.

Transdermal methods, meaning applied to the skin, were

discovered to be effective many years ago. In medical school in the 1960's we were taught that the skin was an impermeable barrier to the 'outside world.' Today, we now know that this is not true. Our skin is an organ that *absorbs*. Today, more and more medicines are being applied to the skin.

With respect to skin absorption of hormones, years ago many French women were showing up at their doctor's and making statements like "I don't understand it; my PMS which used to give me so much trouble has disappeared." Many French doctors heard this story and investigated to find that expensive French skin cream manufacturers were putting hormones in their products. The manufacturers did this because they knew that skin absorbs and that most often a woman's skin is best during pregnancy, when hormone levels are so high.

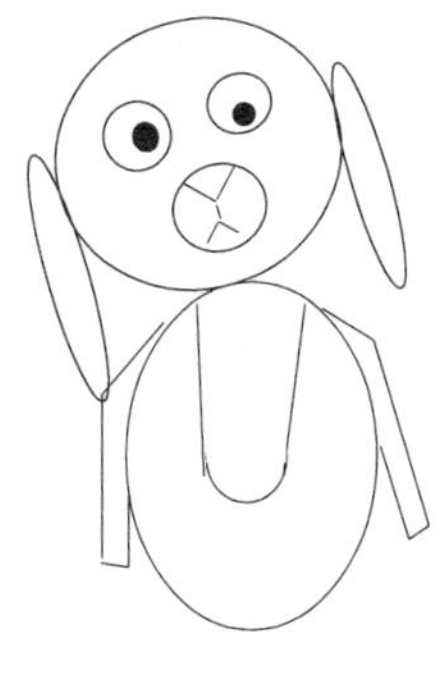

Do you wonder whether or not there are active hormones in the skin preparations? I have a patient who has a female dog that loves to lick. My patient was quite astounded when her older dog, who was spayed when young, became sexually active again (displaying it as dogs do with humans...). Then, as my patient was applying her menopausal hormones to her own legs, she realized that her dog was licking these hormones off of her skin.

Interestingly enough, skin application of hormones more closely mimics the natural distribution process of the body than taking hormones by mouth. Hormones applied to the skin are absorbed and pass directly into the bloodstream. The ovaries, in a biologically similar manner, secrete hormones directly into the bloodstream. The ovarian hormones are distributed to the whole body then eventually wind up in the liver for processing. However, hormones in pill or capsule form given by mouth travel via intestinal lymphatic channels to the liver first, because they are fat-soluble. Here they are biochemically processed, and then distributed to the body via the bloodstream. This phenomenon is called 'first pass through the liver.' Administering hormones through this method is not ideal because it adds to the work of the liver. We believe that direct absorption into the skin more precisely simulates the way the body does it. Sublingual preparations, absorbing through the mucosal surface under the tongue, have this direct absorption advantage as well.

In most, but not all instances, we recommend skin gels. Gels have the added advantage of being beneficial for the skin.

Exceptions exist where capsules taken by mouth and sublingual preparations placed under the tongue are preferred. In one exception, where women have sleep disturbances, we often prescribe oral doses of progesterone at bedtime. We do this because, for unknown reasons, the first pass of progesterone through the liver, prior to distribution via the bloodstream, seems to help sleep disturbance. In other instances, some women do better with the sublingual preparation than with the capsule. Also, as with skin gels, a more finely incremental and precise dose can be achieved with the sublingual preparations.

Titration of Hormones for Proper Dosages

We are ready to consider in general how to determine your optimal dosage of whatever hormone we may choose. The best way to arrive at proper dosage is through utilizing a principle of chemistry called titration. I can more simply describe titration by explaining thyroid hormone dose determination. When we suspect a patient could benefit from thyroid hormone, at the onset of treatment we do not truly know their optimal dose. This is because of differences in individual sensitivity, need and absorption. We have the patient discover their optimal dose. They take one thyroid pill a day for a week. Then they take two pills per day in the second week, three pills per day in the third, and so on until, and if, they reach a six pill-per-day maximum. Our objective is to get two questions answered:

- First, is the hormone an appropriate and beneficial one for the patient. For example, does it alleviate symptoms, and lead to greater well-being?
- And second, if beneficial, at what point is the dose optimal?

Patients often report something similar to the following story of one of our patients:

> "The first week, doc, I didn't notice a thing. The second week I did notice something subtle. The third week I definitely could feel something and I liked it! The fourth week I felt even better on the four pills. The fifth week I felt nervous, hyper, had a tremor, rapid pulse and couldn't sleep! So I went back to four pills a day and felt great again! Four pills are my dose."

Liking the treatment and feeling good are important signs with hormone treatment. Unlike taking vitamins, which can be so subtle that benefits may not be obvious, hormones are not subtle. If they are good for you, you will *like* them. In our example with thyroid hormone, obviously during the dosage of the fifth week, overdose occurred! If you feel funny or strange on your hormones, they either are not proper for you or the dose or preparation is incorrect.

If hormones are good for you, you will like them.

In titration you can reach your optimal dose by incremental increases until you feel symptom alleviation. You can then continue with incremental increases until you feel symptoms of excess. At that point you incrementally decrease your dosage until symptoms of excess are alleviated. There is a very important exception. When dealing with women with risk factors, we may choose to titrate to a level just barely above initial symptom alleviation and stop there (or, we may choose to not use the hormone at all). Finally, after being on the comfortable dose of a hormone a few months, we will often do a lab test to confirm that the dosage levels of the hormones are safe.

Treatment: Optimal Hormones & Dosages, *Progesterone*

Let's continue the subject of treatment with hormones and consider progesterone. Many women benefit from taking progesterone. Treatment can begin during the perimenopausal years and continue throughout your lifetime. Those of you with mood, energy, sleep, or bone issues should consider taking this hormone, as should most every woman. Progesterone can facilitate a dramatic improvement!

I usually recommend using a 3% progesterone gel dispensed by a compounding pharmacy. This needs to be prescribed by a physician. We may change to a 10% gel for a woman that needs a larger amount of progesterone each day. A 10% gel is not that much more expensive than a 3% gel (because the main cost is in the labor of preparation) and it can cover less surface area when larger doses are needed. Many women however will ultimately wind up with excess dosing on a 10% gel. As I mentioned, occasionally we may add or substitute another 25 - 100 mg. of additional progesterone in capsule form at bedtime to treat serious sleep disturbance. We are interested in seeing if sleep disturbance can be ameliorated by progesterone. If it is not, we will look further, because there are other causes and treatments of sleep problems.

How much of the 3% gel to apply to your skin depends on what stage of menopause you are in and on your sensitivity, absorption, and biochemical individuality. With some initial guidelines, utilizing titration, experimentation, and at times, additional guidance, you can usually find your optimal dose. In figure 16 on the next page, you will find symptoms of deficiency and overdose that can be your guideposts in finding your dose. Note that with progesterone, optimal dose will show results in improved sleep, better moods, feeling more relaxed, reduced breast tenderness, decreased water retention, and, if you are still menstruating, a more regular period. Excessive dose can lead to waking up groggy or edgy, a depressed feeling, and water retention. Note that at the bottom of figure 16, there is a

figure 16: Finding Optimal Dose of Progesterone by Symptoms of Inadequacy and Excess

Progesterone deficiency:

sleep problems
breast tenderness
water retention
emotional mood problems, sometimes severe
period irregularities if you are still menstruating

Adequate Progesterone:

Improved sleep
Reduced breast tenderness
Feeling more relaxed, in better mood
Decreased water retention
A more regular period if you are still menstruating

Progesterone Excess:

Drowsiness
Waking up groggy or edgy
Slight dizziness
Increased water retention
Sense of physical instability
Depressed feeling
Feeling of being drunk or spinning
Heaviness of the extremities

Unusual Response to Progesterone:

Antsy, anxious, can't sleep & water retention
[cortisol & deoxycorticosterone are related to the cause]
Hot flashes, or depression [overload of estrogen receptors]
Increased appetite + weight gain [unclear cause]
[Possible increased incidence of Candida Albicans]

list of some rare and unusual progesterone effects. These can occur and can be addressed when they do.

For a woman well into menopause by at least a year or more, we recommend 1/8th to 1/4 teaspoon of 3% progesterone gel applied once or twice daily to the skin in a manner described in figure 21 on page 105. Also refer to figure 17 on page 88 for further guidelines. We want the teaspoon measure to be as accurate as are cooking teaspoons. We use the deficiency and overdose guidelines to achieve or reach optimal dose. As I mentioned, if more than 1/4 tsp. is needed to reach optimal dose we can change to a stronger percent gel so a lesser amount needs to be applied to the skin. Most of the time, women can succeed just as well with a convenient single application put on at night only.

For a woman who is still menstruating yet is experiencing estrogen excess or 'dominant' symptoms, there are different guidelines for administration of progesterone. This woman, in order to counteract her estrogen dominance, will need to modify her progesterone usage following the hormonal patterns of a normal cycle as referred to in the part of figure 3 reproduced on the next page.

We will modify addressing the normal pattern some-

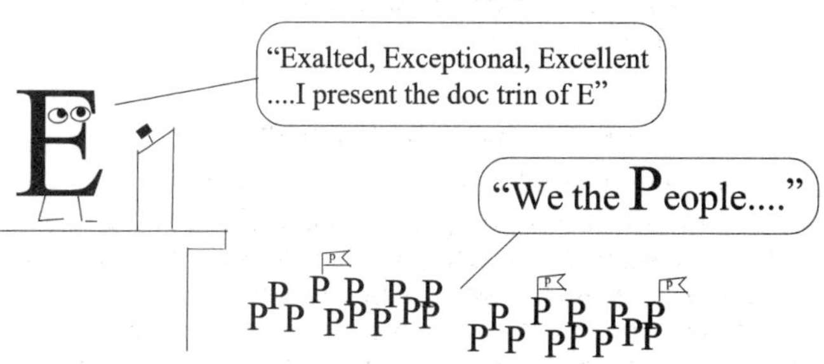

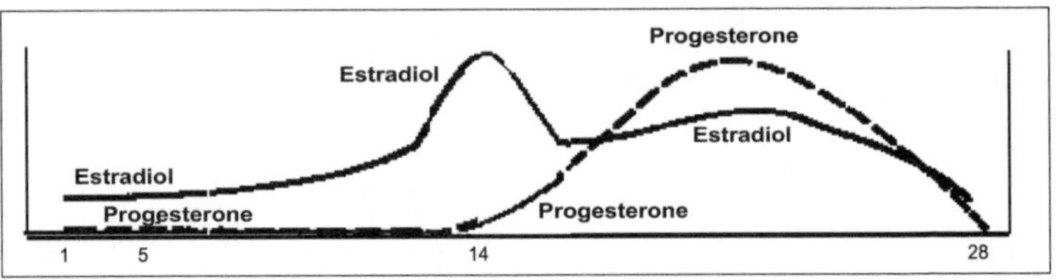

what to deal with the estrogen dominance.

- Begin monthly application of progesterone on day 5, five days after the onset of menstruation.
- Initial dose for day 5 through day 13 can usually be between 1/8th and 1/4 teaspoon, 1 or 2 times/day.
- On day 14, you may want to increase your dose to 1/4 tsp. or more, once or twice daily.
- Be sure to stop applying the gel entirely, on day 28…Stopping progesterone is necessary for you to menstruate.
- Again, exact dosage required for your individual needs will be determined as a result of your 'titration' and experience.
- A single night application is preferable if possible.

If you are still having cycles, be sure to stop using progesterone a day before your expected period...or you may not have one!

As you 'titrate', ask yourself these questions:

- How much will it take to ameliorate estrogen dominant symptoms without getting into progesterone excess symptoms?
- Will your initial doses that work for you be the same ones that you need over time? If you have been progesterone deficient for a long time, initial treatment may also be making up for long-standing deficits. Later evaluation may call for a reduction in dose.

There are other things to consider when titrating progesterone. You may not need to begin monthly supplementation of progesterone until mid-cycle, again following the "normal" estrogen/progesterone pattern as seen on the preceding page.

Should you begin spotting or your period comes earlier than expected, increase progesterone according to guidelines.

- Spotting occasionally when your cycle remains regular can be acceptable. Disregard the spotting and continue taking progesterone. This should regulate you. If it does not, consult your physician.
- Should an unusually heavy flow occur, stop progesterone and consider this day of heavy flow to be the first day of your period. Resume progesterone 5 or 14 days later, according to previous guidelines.
- If your period does not come after stopping progesterone, designate the day you stopped as the first day of your cycle. Start progesterone again in 5 or 14 days.
- At times estrogen dominant symptoms may not be ameliorated after reasonable effort. For one possibility, your liver may not be metabolizing estrogens properly or adequately. In this case estrogen levels build up. Sometimes it is necessary to take measures beyond treatment with progesterone, such as addressing liver function, detoxification, and the excesses of estrogens that have developed.
- Some women do poorly on progesterone! It may not make sense, yet they do not like progesterone at all.

figure 17: Progesterone: Treatment Summary

Progesterone gel 3% 30 mg/g 1 gram = 1/4 tsp
Progesterone capsules 50 or 100 mg strength,
50 - 150 mg additional progesterone
may be needed at night
Progesterone gel 10% sometimes used when
greater amounts of progesterone are needed
Administration in menopause:
1/8th to 1/4 tsp 1 or 2 times daily.
if possible, all at night
possibly additional progesterone in capsule form
for help with sleep disturbance
Administration in perimenopause:
administer in 2nd half of cycle
possibly administer during first half of cycle,
from day 5 to 13
stop taking before your anticipated period
[example: day 28]

- Spotting occasionally when your cycle remains regular can be acceptable. Disregard the spotting and continue taking progesterone. This should regulate you. If it does not, consult your physician.
- Should an unusually heavy flow occur, stop progesterone and consider this day of heavy flow to be the first day of your period. Resume progesterone 5 or 14 days later, according to previous guidelines.
- If your period does not come after stopping progesterone, designate the day you stopped as the first day of your cycle. Start progesterone again in 5 or 14 days.
- At times estrogen dominant symptoms may not be ameliorated after reasonable effort. For one possibility, your liver may not be metabolizing estrogens properly or adequately. In this case estrogen levels build up. Sometimes it is necessary to take measures beyond treatment with progesterone, such as addressing liver function and detoxification.
- Some women do poorly on progesterone! It may not make sense, yet they do not like progesterone at all.

If Hormones Are Right They Feel Right

Again, in administering progesterone, or any other hormone, if the hormones are right for you, they are going to 'feel right' and make you feel good. This is absolute! People who need hormones and take the right ones in the right doses definitely feel better! If you do not feel good from taking hormones, something is definitely wrong and changes need to be made. It is necessary then to get assistance.

There are however, exceptions to what I have just stated! There are women supplementing hormones who feel as if things are fine, yet when we test them they are not fine! This is not common, yet, four such examples are:

- Hormone levels are actually elevated, even though the woman does not have symptoms or signs of excess. This can be revealed by the testing, and in the long run this elevation is not safe.
- Estrogens are not elevated, yet are not being biochemically processed in a preferred and safe way.
- Ovarian hormone production is significantly shut down from use of the birth control pill.
- Other hormones, such as thyroid or adrenal, are diminished and are influencing ovarian hormone function.

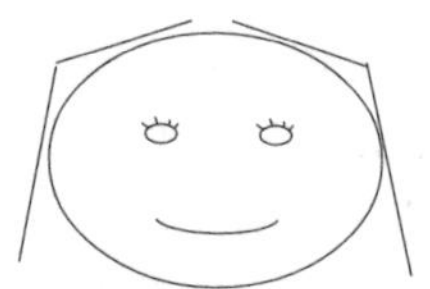

Umm, is that 1/8th tsp in the morning and a pill in the evening?

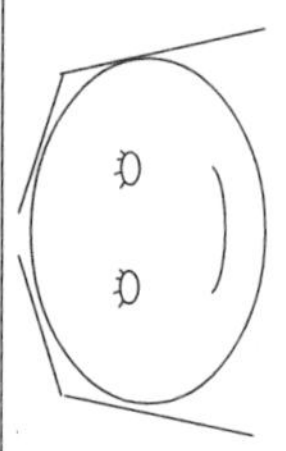

It's hard to believe that our faces look so similar and our doses could be so different

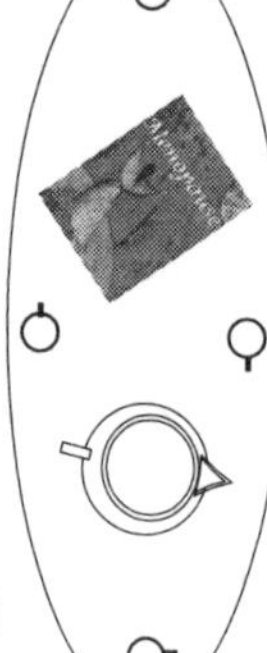

Or is it 1/4 in the morning and 1/8 at night... or 1/4 of 1/8 with a 50mg night cap?

I think I have to apply it on day 3 to 8...or was it on my forehead or is it on my 45th birthday?

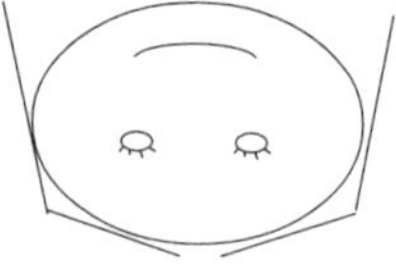

I think I'm going to need to enroll in medical school

Optimal Hormones & Dosages*: Estrogen*

Probably the most complex of the three ovarian hormones to treat and balance are the estrogens. (There is no actual hormone called "estrogen." 'Estrogen' or 'estrogens' —the words are often used interchangeably—are referring to a class of hormones in which there are several *specific* estrogens). As hormones, estrogens are more complex and can be associated with more risk factors. Risks are the primary consideration when determining whether or not to supplement with estrogens in menopause. Excessive or inappropriate estrogens can be associated with a myriad of health problems, some of them serious. The worst risk is cancer of a female organ. For example, breast cancer, like any serious illness, may be caused by a multitude of factors. One of the passible links is to estrogens. Genetics, toxicity, problems of immunity, and many other factors can play a significant role as well. Links need to be respected and analyzed, but links are not absolute cause. For example, if a close female relative has had breast cancer, it does not mean that you are going to get it. This information is considered as a risk factor in your total personal history.

Estrogens are more complex and can be associated with more risk factors.

Six critical subjects to keep in mind when considering the use of estrogens are:

- Chronic over-stimulation of breast, uterus & ovaries from estrogen dominance is unacceptable.

- Inadequate and inappropriate metabolic processing of estrogens by the liver can lead to the lingering presence and effect of excessive and/or more aggressive estrogens.
- The evaluation of faulty estrogen processing may need to include examination of the liver. It may also require evaluation of the intestinal tract for occult infection, which could be a possible source of difficulty for the liver.
- Exposure to and elimination of toxics such as herbicides and pesticides which exist in non-organic foods, and in our environment. These have biological estrogenic effect in the body. They add to the total estrogen effect and can be part of any symptom pattern of estrogen dominance.
- When estrogens are used, bio-identical estrogens that are derived from natural plant sources and which are molecularly-identical to human ovarian hormones is recommended. This includes, in my opinion, not using estrogens derived from synthetic chemicals or from the urine of pregnant horses.
- If there are risk factors related to breast, uterus or ovaries, we recommend that if you use estrogen, you do so only under guidance of a knowledgeable practitioner.
- Special testing can unveil problems with estrogens (see next section).

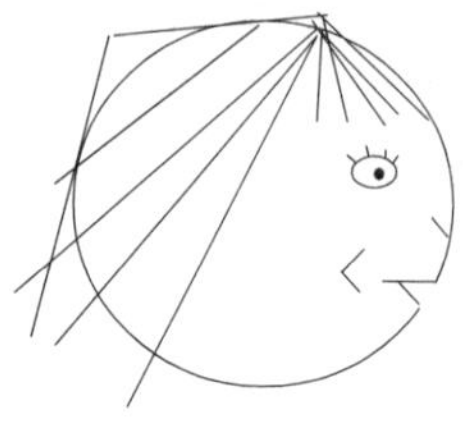

Oh no,
he's doing his
doctor-thing again

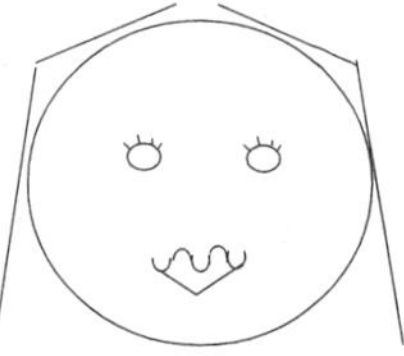

Several of the causes of estrogen dominance, which I have described, are complex. Let's review some of the principle reasons for estrogen dominance:

- Failure of ovulation, which causes lack of progesterone needed to balance estrogen effects.
- Intake of pharmaceutical estrogens, estrogens injected into livestock, and estrogenically active substances derived from the herbicides and pesticides and other compounds contaminating our food.
- Birth control pills.
- Never having been pregnant or having breast-fed an infant.
- Inadequate or incorrect processing of the estrogens in the liver.
- Toxic or intestinal infection problems that have led to liver difficulties.

At times I repeat these subjects for emphasis. Before considering the use of estrogens, we must look at these factors to evaluate and take special measures where advisable.

In the course of treatment, our goal is to avoid estrogen excess, as well as to ameliorate estrogen deficiency. Deficiency can be as significant a problem as inappropriate usage. To reiterate, common symptoms of estrogen deficiency listed in figure 13c on page 65 and figure 18 on page 96, include hot flashes, night sweats, vaginal dryness, difficulty falling asleep, foggy mind, wobbly mood, pain with intercourse, loss of breast fullness… and there are many more. Estrogen deficiency also relates to bone loss and the incidence of heart artery problems.

Once again, careful examination of the details of the individual situation of each woman will usually reveal the safest and best approach to treatment. Many women have come to fear estrogen, as if it were a 'bad' hormone. There have been and are reasons for this fear. However, it is still appropriate to consider estrogen supplementation. It is not wise to summarily disregard estrogen. Some women will need to avoid estrogens and others will benefit from them. With diligent trial and guidance, and with careful consideration of risk factors, we can arrive at a wonderful program that you celebrate for years!

If estrogen is called for in treatment, how do we go about titrating it? As previously discussed, and seen in an excerpt from figure 3 below, in the original estrogen pat-

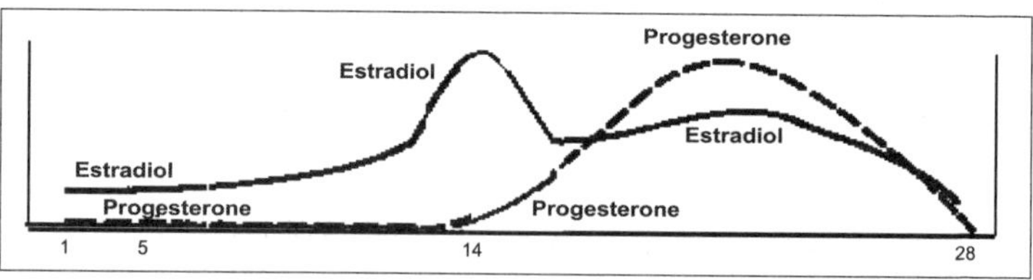

tern in the menstrual cycle, we are reminded that estrogen is excreted throughout most of the cycle. When treating with estrogen, we want to closely replicate this same natural biological pattern. We begin by administering an initial amount of estrogen, estimating on the low side, and watch for its effect. We watch for alleviation of symptoms, such as hot flashes and vaginal dryness. If symptoms are not alleviated in a certain time period, perhaps after several days or a week, we increase the dose. We monitor for symptoms of estrogen excess, such as breast tenderness (especially around the nipple) and water retention. If symptoms of excess develop, we stop the estrogens until the symptoms disappear, then begin again with a lesser dose.

When treating with estrogen, it is very important to also treat with progesterone, either prior to or concurrent with the estrogen. A classic example, that I have given before, occurs in perimenopause. This is a time when your estrogen levels are considerably less than when you were in your twenties. Yet if you do not ovulate, you do not produce adequate progesterone to balance the estrogen that you do have. You might be fooled if you developed an estrogen dominant symptom such as breast tenderness and did not understand the details of what is going on. It is possible to have significantly low estrogen levels, (though still be cycling) yet still have estrogen dominance symptom if there is no progesterone to balance the estrogen. Likewise, if you are supplementing with estrogen, you need adequate progesterone to balance the estrogen. It is important when treating with estrogen to consider the following:

- Take progesterone to balance any pre-existing estrogen dominance, then,
- if it is advisable to treat with estrogen, determined primarily by risk factor and need considerations, adjust the progesterone to balance additional estrogen.

To help you titrate and monitor estrogen supplementation, you can find a short list of symptoms of excess estrogen in figure 18 on the next page. Common symptoms of excess are breast tenderness (and enlargement), water retention (that you can discover if your rings are too tight), and, irritability, yet with a clear mind. Breast tenderness is discovered earliest by putting pressure on the area of your nipples.

figure 18:
Finding Optimal Dose of Estrogen by Symptoms of Inadequacy and Excess

Inadequate:

Hot flashes
Vaginal dryness
Loss of breast fullness, drooping
Sleep disturbance: difficulty falling asleep, with restlessness, night sweats
Weight gain, especially in hips, thighs & buttox
Mind foggy in the morning,
Feeling a "little down"
Confused, not in good control of your mood

Excess:

Breast tenderness, especially in nipple area
Water retention, rings too tight
Feeling uptight, irritated, yet with a clear mind
Breast fullness, growing

When treating with estrogens, the symptoms from deficiency can often respond quite rapidly. For example, you might be right in the midst of a hot flash, apply an estrogen skin gel, and have the hot flash go away in minutes. When you get skilled with timing and dosage you should be able to quiet down some estrogen deficiency symptoms rapidly and then eliminate them in the long run. However, should you overdose with estrogens and wind up with breast tenderness for example, it can take days or longer to quiet down the symptom even after stopping the estrogen supplementation.

In treating with estrogens, we most commonly recommend a preparation known as 'bi-est' that is applied to the skin. It is derived ultimately from soy. It contains 2 major estrogens, estradiol and estriol, and is prepared by compounding pharmacists. For a background to understanding this, you can see in figure 2 on page 23 that biochemically, estradiol, abbreviated 'E2,' and estrone, 'E1,' derive from testosterone. They are the most potent of the estrogens. 'Estriol' or 'E3,' which is different from estradiol, is produced from the metabolism of estrone. Estriol is a significantly weaker estrogen, which achieves its highest levels in pregnancy. Estriol has a major beneficial effect on the vagina during pregnancy. It prepares the vaginal tissue for childbirth. Research cited earlier indicates sufficient levels of estriol may be 'cancer-protective.' Later studies have revealed that the estrogen metabolism picture is more complex, and we will address it.

In treating with estrogens, my preference is a 2.75 mg./gram of a 'Bi-est' preparation in a hydro-alcoholic skin gel (called 'carbopol') base. Bi-est contains 2 mg./gram of estriol as well as 0.75 mg./g of estradiol, thus present in a 2.67 to 1 ratio. This formulation does not contain estrone. I recommend not including estrone in an estrogen preparation because of information derived from 24 hour urine hormone tests of estrogens in menopausal women. In these tests we consistently find very low levels of estradiol and estriol, yet consistently normal or elevated levels for estrone. This estrone is present in these amounts because it is produced in fat tissue (wow! produced in fat tissue!) and its production does not rely on the ovaries or the adrenal glands. There is no reason to include estrone in any preparation. Some women seem to do better on tri-est, which contains all 3 of the above estrogens. In general, I still recommend that most women who are on a popular product called 'tri-est,' switch to bi-est. Many women on tri-est when tested, prove to have excessive levels of estrone. Precise treatment regarding this can be ascertained from proper hormone testing.

The amount of bi-est to apply depends again upon titration. You can either wait until you have titrated progesterone to optimal levels, or if symptomatic, you can begin the bi-est at the same time as the progesterone. Initially you can apply the bi-est gel to the skin at bedtime, especially if hot flashes or sweating are keeping you up at night. If daytime hotflashes remain a problem, you may want to apply an extra dose in the morning. It is common to begin with a low dose, such as 1/8th teaspoon once daily.

Compounding pharmacists also supply this gel in a tube. A common equivalent to 1/8th tsp. is 1 inch of gel squeezed out onto your hand (providing concentrations in the tube are equivalent to concentrations in a jar). Check with your pharmacist. If you are still menstruating, you might start application on day 5 of your cycle. If you are no longer menstruating you can apply that amount every day.

Remember to not apply estrogens to the front of your torso. Here, I am describing the region between the bottom of your neck and top of your pubic bone, and between your shoulders. We do not want direct estrogen stimulation to the breasts, thus avoid application and absorption in this region. Once again, the goal is to achieve a balance between alleviating estrogen deficiency symptoms and avoiding estrogen excess symptoms. These symptoms are listed in abbreviated form in figure 18 on page 96. Also refer to figure 19 on the next page for information summarizing treatment. (All hormone figures are repeated in 'Summary.')

figure 19:
Estrogen Treatment Summary

Bi-est Gel:
Do not apply to the front of the torso
2.75 mg/gram = 0.75 mg/g Estradiol [E2], 2 mg/g Estriol [E3]
1/8th tsp = 0.5 gram, 1/4 tsp = 1 gram
Common starting dose: Apply 1/8th tsp 1 or 2 times/day
increase dosages by 1/16th tsp
[1/2 of 1/8th tsp] if necessary
If you have night sweats, increase the night dose.
Adjust, adjust, adjust!
If menstruating, begin on day 5, end on day 28, and
follow the 'estrogen menstrual curve' [figure 3]
If possible, you may be able to consolidate to a
single, nightly dose.

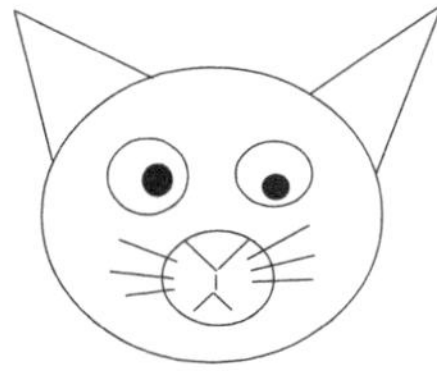

The plot is about to thicken

Estrone Metabolism: the 'Handling' of Estrogens and Risk

On a final note regarding estrogens and estrogen risk, I am going to guide you through another way to reduce risks when working with estrogens. Research continues to unravel the association of estrogen with the huge rise in the incidence of breast and other female cancers. (Remember, there is a lot more to cancer than just estrogens). Recall that once produced, the body degrades and eliminates estrogens as it does all hormones. The whole process is dependent upon the health of the liver and the intestine.

Research has unveiled that there are aggressive, gene-toxic and more dangerous estrogens. These toxic estrogens result from the poor biochemical handling of estrone. In figure 20a below, you will find an expanded version of the biochemical roadmap first presented in figure 2 on page 23. Look in the lower right hand corner at figure 20a. Here we have roadmaps on the processing of the estrogens. What you need to know is that the faulty processing of estrogens is part of the problem found with the rise in the incidence of breast cancer, when estrogens are part of the cause. Consider the following (and refer to the inset of figure 20a re-

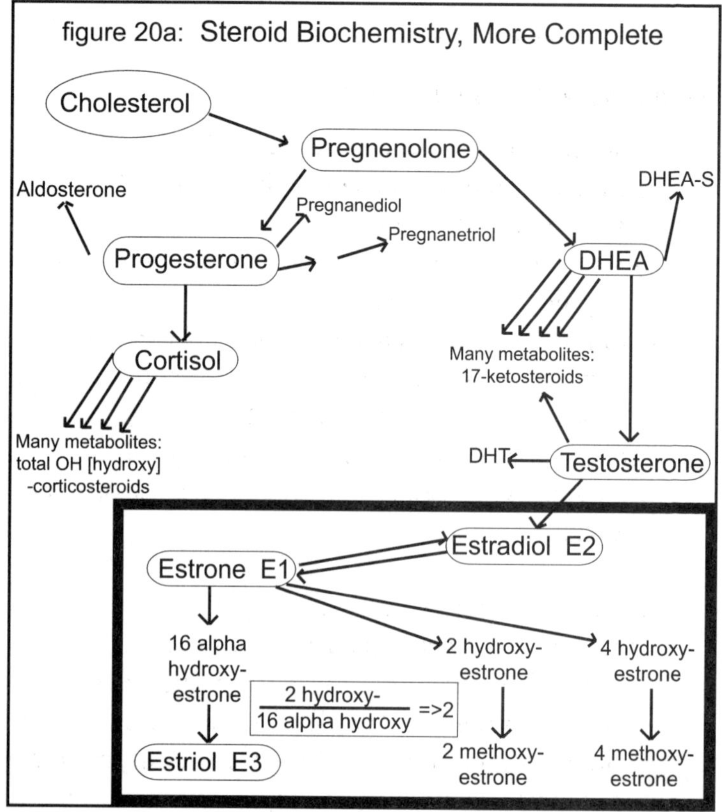

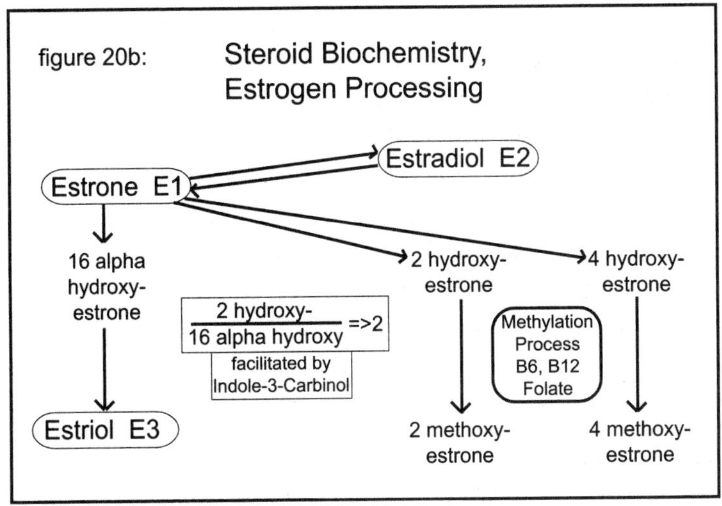

produced above as figure 20b):

- Estrone is produced from estradiol.
- Estrone is handled biochemically in steps. These steps are called 'pathways.'
- Estrone can be handled in 3 different ways, travelling down 3 different pathways.
- No matter which pathway it takes, the estrone first converts into intermediary products and then those products convert into end products.
- Of the estrone metabolites, 4 hydroxyestrone is the most toxic. 16 alphahydroxy estrone is the next most toxic.

In the conversion we want 2 things to happen.

- Number 1, we want all conversions to go all the way to the final end products and not linger in the intermediary products. We don't want lingering in the intermediary products because the intermediary products are more toxic. Again, the most toxic of the estrone intermediate products is the 4 hydroxy. The second most toxic is the 16 alpha hydroxy.

- Secondly, it matters which pathway the estrone takes because one pathway is safer than the others. The 2 hydroxy-to-methoxy pathway is the safest. The estriol pathway is the next safest.

I am emphasizing this because safety in augmenting estrogens is of prime importance. When considering handling estrogens in the liver, once again we find that significant health issues in menopause can go beyond the ovarian hormones to include the health of other systems of the body.

We can uncover details of the risks I have mentioned through special testing. We like to do this with as many women as possible and especially in situations where a woman's medical story reveals increase in risk. Sometimes we wait until a woman has discovered her optimal doses on bi-est and then test. We do this in preference to testing prior to treatment in a woman who is menopausal, whose estrogen levels would be very low, thus testing would not reveal adequate information regarding her ability to process estrogens.

We can influence all of these biochemical estrogen processing risks in a favorable way (see figure 20b pg 101) by:

- Addressing underlying intestinal or liver problems, if indicated.
- Supplementing with:
  * Vitamin B 12 in a sublingual, hydroxy or methyl cobalamin form, approximately 2000 micrograms per day

* Folic acid, approximately 5 mg. per day
* Vitamin B 6, approximately 50 mg. per day
* Indole-3-carbinol, (which is present in vegetables such as broccoli and brussel sprouts, and is also available as a nutritional supplement. I recommend 400 mg. per day.

These supplements and the assistance they give to the proper processing of estrogens, can be quite profound in their effect. Clinical trials in a group of women with severe PMS, which is primarily due to excess estrogens, demonstrated major reduction of symptoms from taking the supplements listed above. Again, these supplements are designed to help properly process estrogens and reduce them.

It all may sound complex, yet in the long run, it isn't difficult. Ultimately you will be applying a few gels and taking nutritional supplements. The same supplements that help you process estrogens also happen to help you process another substance called homocysteine which is a major preventive measure for arteriosclerosis. Thus the benefit of this program can be far reaching.

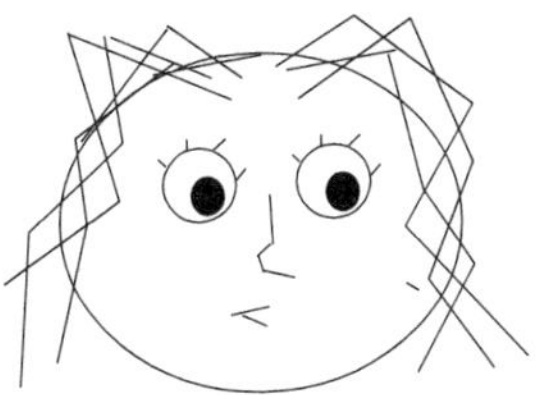

I'm not stressed
by menopause,
are you?

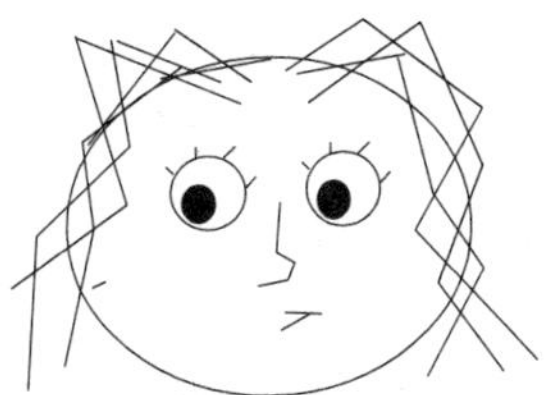

Menopause
Schmenopause!

Method of Application of Skin Gels

Let's take a moment to discuss general strategies of application of skin gels. In most cases, for practicality, we recommend once daily application. We consider hydroalcoholic gel preparations with minimal alcohol content to be the best. At times twice daily application is needed.

We suggest that you carefully measure out your dose onto your hands and begin the first night by applying it to your feet and ankles. The next time you apply it, apply where you left off, to your lower legs. And again, the next time, apply where you left off, perhaps to the knees and thighs. You continue on up your body until you reach your face. Then, start all over again at your feet.

No matter where you are applying estrogen or progesterone on your body, each time, save a tiny bit in your hands for application to your face, neck and back of the hands. These hormones are good for your skin and these areas are the most vulnerable parts of skin.

There are notable exceptions:

- Do not apply estrogen preparations to the front of your torso. We do not want direct estrogen stimulation of your breasts.
- You *can* apply progesterone gel to your breasts. For women with fibrocystic breast disease, we often prescribe a stronger progesterone gel and have them apply it twice daily to breasts alone.
- Do not apply testosterone to your face, front of torso, or to hairy areas of your skin. You could cause acne or facial hair growth, or excessive hair growth in

already hairy areas.

- If you are applying more than one hormone, and happen to forget where you had applied one of them the night before, do not be concerned. Just start over again on your feet.

figure 21: Hormone Treatment, General Information

Types of Hormones:

Pill/Capsules

compounded capsules,
synthetic estrogens, Premarin, Provera, PremPro, Birth Control pill

Skin preparations:

compounded creams & gels, patches

Sublingual preparations

Skin gels in general:

Apply before bedtime and in the morning
Exception:
You may find that you can do just as well with one application of gels per day, for convenience..& best at night

Apply starting with feet & ankles, then legs, then knees and thighs, etc until you reach 'the top' [your neck]...then begin again
Exception:
save a little for your face, neck & back of hands every time
Exception:
Do not apply estrogens to the front of your torso [neck to pubic area, and between your shoulders]
Exception:
Do not apply testosterone to the front of your torso or to face or to hairy areas of your body

Hydroalcoholic base is best
Bi-est for skin,
Estriol &/or testosterone vaginal gel for vagina if indicated
[available also in a non-hydroalcoholic gel]

Treatment with Hormones: Testosterone

Testosterone is another important hormone to consider for a woman going through menopause. Figure 22 on the next page lists testosterone deficiency symptoms. These include diminished libido, diminished energy and stamina, diminished sense of security, hair loss, flabbiness, and muscular weakness, especially of the upper arms and cheeks. Again, if and how much of this hormone you might need depends on what your body has been used to, and how much production of this hormone you have lost! I recommend trying testosterone under these conditions:

- if your symptoms or tests suggest a need for it
- after you found an optimal program of progesterone, and, if applicable, bi-est.

The titration of testosterone follows the same protocol as with other hormones:

- titrate up to optimal dose based on the inadequate and excess symptoms summarized in figure 22 on the next page. Excess testosterone leads to excessive aggressiveness, an excessive oiliness of the skin, acne, and hair growth where you have applied it, or on the face.
- Realize that you may have to adjust progesterone and/ or estrogen dosages once introducing testosterone. This may be necessary because of all of the biochemical interrelationships of these hormones.

For testosterone, I also recommend a hydro-alcoholic gel, 4mg/gram, beginning with 1/8th teaspoon applied once or twice daily, and not applied to face or hairy areas or the front of the torso. For some vaginal conditions such as a more severe atrophic form of vaginitis, there are also special non-alcoholic preparations of testosterone that can be used, along with estriol in a vaginal gel.

figure 22: Finding Optimal Dose of Testosterone by Symptoms of Inadequacy and Excess

Inadequate:	*Excess:*
Diminished libido	Hyper aggressiveness
Loss of sense of security	Hair growth in unwanted places eg. face, and where gel is applied
Diminished energy and stamina	Acne
Flabbiness & Muscular weakness; upper arms, cheeks	Excessive oiliness of skin
Hair loss	

Important Variations and Alternatives

Having stated these basic guidelines, know that there are many individual variations and exceptions possible. There are women who need to apply hormones twice daily. There are women that need to apply more bi-est at night to control night-time hot flashes and sleep disturbance. There are women that need a stronger bi-est. There are women that benefit from additional estriol for the vagina and at times we recommend a direct vaginal preparation with a non-alcoholic base. There are women who also benefit from testosterone for vaginal application. There are women that prefer capsules or sublingual drops. There are women that feel awful on any estrogen. There are some women where excessive progesterone use can lead to estrogen dominant symptoms through the 'unusual progesterone effect,' (summarized in figure 16 on page 84). There are women that feel awful on any progesterone. The exceptions go on and on.

We can develop good ideas regarding your taking hormones, yet ultimately the "proof is in the pudding." We know that when a woman feels better we are close, to or have reached, an optimal hormone treatment program. There are circumstances when "feeling better" also needs to be confirmed with proper testing, to make sure we are not using excessive doses, or that estrogens are being handled properly.

It is very significant that there have been many women who have passed into and through menopause and have taken nothing at all, and have had no problems at all. There are also many women who prefer not to supplement hormones and can still achieve satisfying or excellent results from using diet, nutritional supplements, and herbs for menopause. Many good doctors and practitioners have other approaches that they prefer. Conversely, many women do not succeed with these approaches alone.

The possible use of herbs for the treatment of menopause raises another question. Herbs are molecules that are non-identical to those in our body, and thus technically are 'medicines.' The body integrates identical molecules (such as foods) yet *reacts* to the non-identical. It is this reaction that we capitalize on for medicinal effect. Use of any medicine, including herbs, is best done for an impeccable period of time, which most often, should not be long range. Herbs therefore may not be ideally suited for the treatment of menopause.

So what is the best approach for you? Once again it will all come down to your individual situation with all of your details, your risks, your preferences, your intuition and knowing...your wise choice!

Chapter Eleven
Testing

Are there other ways to know if you need treatment for menopause besides experiencing obvious, self-evident and uncomfortable symptoms in your body? Terrific tests are available to provide high-resolution views of hormonal levels. There are also numerous fundamental methods to assess female health that are relevant and important, some of which are enumerated in figure 23 below.

figure 23: **Testing**

Self Breast Exam

Breast and Pelvic exam with Pap smear
by a trained practitioner

Pelvic ultrasound
for endometrial lining, uterus, and ovaries.

Hormone Tests

Other, specialized Gynecologic and other testing
based on indications + risk/benefit
including mammogram, bone density,
and other tests and procedures

Hormonal Testing

Testing for hormones is valuable, interesting, and sometimes crucial to a successful treatment program. For the purpose of saving money, testing can be bypassed in many instances with no significant adverse consequences. However, when initial attempts at rational treatments do not succeed, or significant risk factors for breast, uterine or ovarian problems exist, testing is very important.

There are 3 principle methods of hormone testing and the methods are based upon sample collection of blood, saliva or urine. Each method has its advantages and disadvantages. Most practitioners have their preferred methods of testing and their favorite laboratories. By observing results over time, a practitioner will learn a great deal about hormones and how lab results correlate with individual patients and their symptoms. This level of practical experience over a significant amount of time is crucial. In understanding and interpreting laboratory tests, nothing will replace the personal experience of an individual health practitioner using reasonable methods and good laboratories in the long-term process of testing and correlating lab results with many of their patients.

My preferred method in most cases of testing hormones is a 24 hour urine collection with a specific laboratory in California (AAL). I prefer the 24 hour urine test because hormone levels fluctuate in a 24 hour period. Samples taken over a 24 hour period can be more representative than blood and saliva samples that are taken from one moment in time. This method also affords us the opportunity to examine the *metabolic byproducts* of the hormones, as well as principle hormones. Metabolic byproducts reflect actual hormonal utilization, rather than just hormone presence. They also provide us with a tool to assess risk of illness.

The 24 hour test must be obtained through a licensed health practitioner. The test evaluates the urine for levels of (see figure 20a on page 100):

- Progesterone: through 2 metabolic byproducts
- Estrogens: the three major ones, E1 estrone, E2 estradiol, and E3 estriol
- Estrogen processing metabolites: 5 of them, to assess safety of estrogen processing
- Testosterone
- Thyroid hormones: T4 & T3
- Adrenal hormones: 5 major hormones and 8 of their processed byproducts
- Growth hormone
- Minerals: sodium, potassium, calcium, magnesium and phosphorous.

There is great advantage in testing all of these hormones together. As I have mentioned earlier, it can be difficult to balance the ovarian hormones if there is significant adrenal or thyroid depletion as well. You could have a hard time achieving menopausal goals with menopausal hormones if the thyroid and adrenals are not addressed concurrently.

There is great advantage in testing adrenal, thyroid and ovarian hormones together.

There are logistics involved in this urine testing. A full 24 hour collection is required. The correct time that we test is also important:

- In a woman that is menstruating we would choose the day that is 3/4's through her cycle. If, for example, she has a 28 day cycle, we would collect on day 20-21, counting day 1 from the first day of menses. This is the time when we can get the optimal information about both estrogen and progesterone, when they have a simultaneous peak in levels in the monthly cycle, as can be seen in the excerpt from figure 3 below.

- If a woman's periods have become irregular, we select the collection day the best we can.

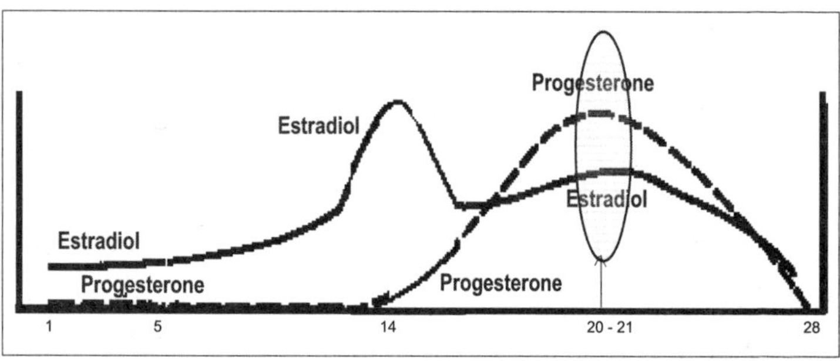

- If menstruation is very irregular, it is difficult to trust accuracy of the ovarian hormones. We do not know what day in the cycle we are sampling and could be measuring one of the lowest of progesterone or estrogen days (figure 3 above). Sometimes with this situation it is preferable to regulate hormonal balance through titration as suggested by symptoms, as previously described, and test after achieving balance to check that levels are reasonable and that estrogens are processed safely.
- If menstruation has ceased, at least for several months, it usually does not matter what day we choose to test. Again, as above, it may be preferable to test after hormone balance is achieved. Again, full into menopause, a woman's estrogens may be too low to assess quality of estrogen processing.
- Incidentally, if you are supplementing hormones now,

even premarin, there is no need to suspend taking them to obtain the test, so long as there has been consistency in taking them, preferably for six weeks. Sometimes it is preferable to change to natural hormone and then test.

- If there is significant liver or kidney disease, 24 hour urine is not an optimal method of testing.

Often we want to test *after* treatment has been established, or changed over to, and stabilized. An example of this is when bi-est is instituted. In more straightforward situations, when hormone treatment proceeds quite easily, if we haven't tested prior to treatment, possibly for financial reasons, we like to do the 24 hour urine test six months into implementation of the bi-est. We can then assess overall hormone levels and balance, as well as learn whether or not the estrogens are being processed properly and safely. Again, we consider this to be particularly important if a woman has risk factors. Also, if a woman is well into menopause, has not yet begun treatment, and is going to use estrogens, we will best learn how she is processing her estrogens when treatment has been well established for awhile and she is at her preferred estrogen dosage.

Testing saliva or blood for hormones is preferred by many practitioners. Both of these methods definitely have their advocates. There are advantages and disadvantages to all methods but I prefer not to use the saliva test in perimenopause or menopause for several reasons:

- Saliva is not a fluid that is part of the normal physiological hormonal circuitry.
- Amounts of hormone in saliva are very small. The amounts are a fraction of that found in blood or urine

and are therefore technically difficult to measure.

- Ovarian hormones in a menopausal woman compared to a younger woman are present in very small amounts and, because of this, are even more difficult to test. Of the hormones that we are considering, only the adrenal hormones DHEA and cortisol are present in relatively larger amounts and thus are easier to test in saliva.
- There are other problems with saliva. I have seen discrepancies in the results in concurrent testing with saliva and urine, with the clinical picture correlated to the urine test.
- Newer testing methods with saliva are currently being evaluated as this book goes to print. Salivary methods may be in the process of improving.

Saliva can be very useful for testing estradiol and progesterone levels in a younger woman where the quantities of these hormones are more ample. In questions of fertility or ovulation, samples can be conveniently collected every three days. This helps us understand hormonal balance throughout the menstrual cycle and indirectly reveals if ovulation is taking place.

Blood testing can sometimes be appropriate for assessing certain aspects of hormones. For example, thyroid blood tests are valuable for uncovering thyroid disease, however they are inadequate when it comes to revealing a 'tired' thyroid gland producing less than optimal hormone levels. Also, though severe adrenal disease can be revealed by blood tests, adrenal fatigue may not be discovered in simple blood testing. Adrenal hormone secretion can fluctuate over a 24 hour period. One can be misled with a normal morning blood cortisol level. The adrenals may be in good enough shape to produce a normal level overnight, yet be too tired to keep up production all day. An afternoon blood sampling for cortisol, which is logistically cumbersome to accomplish, would reveal a low cortisol level in this case. Blood testing of the ovarian hormones can be quite good in the hands of the experienced.

When trying to follow hormone levels in women who are taking hormones, we must be very specific about the time that we test with blood and saliva testing, and then consistently retest at that time. The reason for that is that a hormone pill, when absorbed into your body, reaches peak blood levels over a specific time, and then tapers off. The blood or saliva test result is completely influenced by the time you took your hormones in relationship to the time you take the sample. This is not a problem when assessing a full 24 hour urine and is another reason why I prefer this method.

I believe at this juncture, though I have not exhausted the topic and details of hormonal testing methods, I have given you enough information to consider. Once again, there are advantages and disadvantages to all methods. I definitely have my strong preferences. The knowledge, interest and experience of the individual practitioner are crucial to the choices he or she makes about the methods of testing and the choice of the laboratory.

For the sake of your biochemical entertainment, or, if you should ever have this 24 hour urine hormone test performed, I am including, without further explanation, in figure 24 on the next page, an even more complete biochemi-

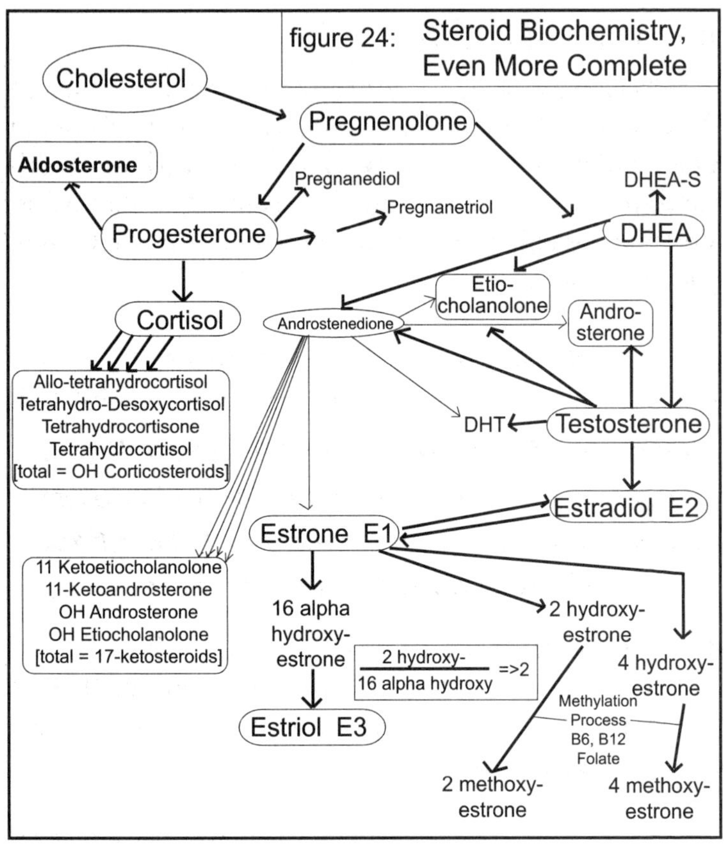

cal roadmap of the steroid hormones that you have come to know and love.

In questions of mood that do not easily resolve, or weight gain, even more testing can be valuable. We are able to assess neurotransmitter levels: norepinephrine, epinephrine, dopamine and serotonin, which can relate closely to problems of weight and mood. Even of more fundamental use is the exploration of glucose, insulin, triglycerides, and cholesterol as they relate to weight and risk. I will have more to say about this.

Basic Female Assessment

There are fundamentals in female medicine for which there is no substitute. These include frequent self-breast exam and periodic breast and pelvic exam by an experienced practitioner. There are many sources for correct instruction for self-breast exam, including pamphlets from your practitioner's office.

I would like to add two suggestions for your breast health. The first is to diminish bra-wearing time. Medical studies have strongly identified the value of this. This allows for freer circulation of the lymphatic drainage fluid in the lymph vessels for the natural removal of toxic, metabolic and other wastes.

There are fundamentals in female medicine: frequent breast self-exam and periodic breast and pelvic exam by an experienced practitioner. There is no substitute for them.

The second is simple massage, easily performed in your shower or bath, that helps lymphatic drainage in the breasts. Stabilize a breast at the nipple with the fingers of one hand. With the fingers of your other hand, press firmly near the nipple and move out peripherally, continuing to firmly press to the edge of the breast. Repeat this 'milking-type' process from center to edge, until you have

Reduced bra-wearing time and breast lymphatic drainage self-massage can make a major difference in breast health.

covered all the area of both breasts. Lymphatic channels are low-pressure drainage vessels. Assisting fluid movement within them by external massage is very beneficial from time to time.

Although the vast majority of breast and pelvic exams reveal no problems, occasionally something is uncovered. Ideally this would happen at an early stage where further evaluation, intervention and treatment can make a beneficial and crucial difference. Evaluation and testing of this nature is important and can be critical.

Ultrasound is another testing method that can have great merit. Information gained from this non-invasive technique that utilizes a low intensity of energy can reveal an ovarian cyst or tumor, a breast abnormality, a uterine fibroid, and even a thickened endometrial lining.

Breast diagnosis by thermography is being evaluated for efficacy. In theory it holds significant promise, yet to me, it is far too early to feel confident about it's accuracy.

There are other more invasive tests available which we need to assess and weigh carefully against the indications and risks involved. I would put mammograms and bone densitometry in this category. There are also cases where mammography and bone density tests are quite important. In my opinion, these tests should not be unequivocally included as 'routine' nor categorically dismissed .

Your gynecologist also has many other examinations and tests for evaluation and treatment that can be very important.

Chapter Twelve
Osteoporosis

No discussion of menopause would be complete without including the subject of osteoporosis. Osteoporosis is bone loss, sometimes mild (osteopenia), sometimes severe enough to cause too-easy fracture of a hip. Osteoporosis has as many factors associated with its development as does bone itself…and bone is quite alive, dynamic and complex! In examining the causes of and treatments for osteoporosis, we will consider hormones, nutrition and digestion, buffering of excessive body acid, and exercise.

Our hormones, progesterone, estrogens, and testosterone as well as DHEA and thyroid, play a major role in bone health. Many women have osteoporosis because of hormone deficiency. Any woman with osteoporosis, at a minimum, should be on progesterone. Progesterone directly and beneficially effects cells called osteoblasts which lay down new bone. Estrogen too, needs consideration, however, and of course, with special attention paid to its risk factors. Estrogen slows down the activity of cells called osteoclasts. These cells effect the process that breaks bone down!

Osteoporosis has many factors associated with its development, including insufficient hormones, nutrition and digestion, excessive body acid and inadequate exercise.

From the standpoint of nutrition, bone is made out of protein and minerals. This makes bone subject to the content of these nutrients in the food you purchase and eat. In the past, people often had more nutritious diets. Also they were more physically active and were exposed to less toxins. A healthier diet, exercise and life greatly impacts risk for osteoporosis and other problems.

Most food in America is grossly low in nutrient content. In the 1930's the United States Senate reported that American soils had deficiencies in minerals! Agribusiness has aggravated this situation through unhealthy farming methods. A recent Rutgers University study shows that conventional grocery store fruits and vegetables contain 15% of the minerals found in 'organic' produce from health food stores. Thus, at worst we get 15% (of some already lowered percentage) of the minerals we need! This nutrient content deficiency is the principle reason for the flatter taste in conventional food.

In the 1930's the United States Senate reported that American soils had deficiencies in minerals!

I used to wonder why grocery market food did not taste like food! When I was young my grandparents would take me with them when they would go to pick fresh corn, tomatoes and other produce from a local farm. The taste of the produce was amazing, as was that of chicken and most everything else. What has happened?! Today food can be as bland as the styrofoam it is packaged in! So, the initial problem with respect to bone nutrition can be inadequate nutrient content of the food.

Bone health is also subject to your ability to digest, absorb, and assimilate nutrients that are present in the food.

Digestion is paramount. Digestion begins with chewing. Many people rush through their meals without adequately breaking down food into the tiny particles so important for the subsequent stages of digestion, the kind of tininess that results from competent chewing. Also, natural and fresh foods have actual digestive enzymes in them that assist in their own digestion. Most modern, non-organic foods are grossly deficient in these enzymes.

Bone health is also subject to your ability to digest, absorb and assimilate nutrients that are present in the food.

Additionally, through long-term stress, we have less and less hydrochloric acid, which is necessary for the digestion of protein and minerals in food. Rushing, without chewing, results in insufficient reduction of the particle size of food, which overtaxes the already reduced levels of hydrochloric acid. Also, we have less and less of our own digestive enzymes, which are needed to further digest the elements of food. Hence the amount of digestion of minerals and protein needed and available for our bones is compromised.

Absorption is yet another facet of digestion which effects bone. For a variety of reasons there are widespread intestinal problems, many of which result from hidden, often not readily apparent infections with yeasts, amoeba, worms and/or unbeneficial bacteria. These germs are unacceptable to our immune system. The interaction between our immune system and the infection leads to low-grade inflammation of our intestinal lining. This can lead to gut surface absorptive problems, "leaky gut," "food allergy," and ultimately, to compromised absorption and reduced assimilation of nutrients. Once again, this will result in a reduction of protein and minerals available to the bone rebuilding process.

Overall body acidity is another important factor in osteoporosis. Here, I am referring to acid that can be produced in our cells, and may get excessive from a variety of causes: I am not referring to the stomach acid related to digestion. The bottom line with excessive cellular acidity is that it needs to be neutralized, or 'buffered.' When brittle diabetics end up in emergency rooms it is usually because of excessive acidity. In their case though, that acidity developed from problems related to diabetes. The common and widespread excess acidity we find in many people, is in no way severe or of such immediate threat as it is in diabetic acidosis. Yet, in the long run, problems can be significant from excessive acidity, including problems that can develop from loss of bone minerals. If we have too much acidity, our body must 'buffer,' and it resorts to extracting minerals from bone to neutralize the excess acid!

Our most immediate buffering mechanism combines the acid with bicarbonate present in our blood and this produces carbon dioxide. The carbon dioxide is then exhaled out of our lungs. When this primary mechanism is overloaded from excessive acidity, we utilize a backup buffering system. In this case our body buffers the excessive acid by combining the acid with minerals.

Where does our body acquire the needed minerals to do this type of buffering? From where these minerals are present in greatest abundance: our bones! Our precious bone calcium, magnesium and trace minerals will be extracted from bone, if need be, to address the biological priority of buffering excessive acid.

How do we get too much cellular acid? Food and stress are the two major sources. During the biochemical processing of all foods, on a cellular level, there is the possibility that acid can be produced. This is more probable for some foods than others. Acid forms more from the cellular 'burning' of protein derived from animal food and especially when dietary intake of animal protein is excessive. The other, and usually more significant, producer of excessive cellular acidity is the biochemistry that results from stress! Once again we meet up with another consequence of stress: we see the effect of stress on bone health, just as we have seen it affect hormonal health.

The demand to buffer acid is strong because many of our essential internal biochemicals can be injured by excessive acidity. In our office, we ask most menopausal women, especially anyone with diminished bone density, to test every urination for 2-3 days with an acid-testing paper. If their urines come up too acidic, we make dietary and other adjustments to buffer this excessive acid and therefore conserve bone minerals!

Address the biological priority of buffering excessive acid, so that our precious calcium, magnesium and trace minerals will not be extracted from bone.

Priorities in the treatment of Osteoporosis.

- The program begins with nutrition, which is founded upon food that is organic, organic, organic!
- Protein intake needs to be generous, though not excessive, and the amount can vary according, once again, to a metabolic individuality.
- Digestion needs to be supplemented with proper chewing and digestive enzymes. When tolerated, we also add hydrochloric acid in the form of a dietary supplement called 'betaine hydrochloride.'
- Intestinal absorption and infection issues may need to be addressed.
- Vitamins and Minerals should be supplemented, emphasizing quality mineral supplements in assimilatable form,
    * such as calcium citrate (e.g: 400mg elemental calcium as a citrate) and magnesium glycenate, (e.g: 300 - 600mg elemental magnesium as a glycenate), boron, and other trace minerals,
    * as well as special vitamins, such as D & K, that relate strongly to bone health.
- Hormones, especially progesterone should be customized.
- Acidity should be checked for and adjusted if need be, with diet, and supplements designed to buffer excessive acid.
- And weight bearing exercise such as walking is essential.

obviously!

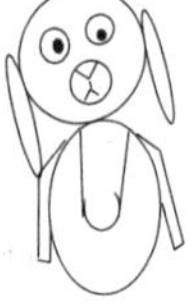

We think dem bones are very important

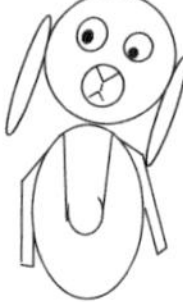

absolutely!

Chapter Thirteen

Weight Issues in Menopause

Weight gain is a common complaint of women at menopause. It also is a complex subject, with many issues related to it. As important as calorie counting and fat intake are, rarely is weight just a matter of these factors. Several biological wear and tear phenomena relate to body weight, and these intersect during a woman's 40's and 50's. These include:

- intake of excessive amounts of carbohydrates, especially simple carbohydrates: 'worst case,' sweets.
- diminished ability to physiologically manage carbohydrates: glucose regulating issues.
- increased insulin resistance caused by excessive carbohydrates, excessive adrenaline, cortisol, glucagon, and diminished estrogens.
- diminished neurotransmitter levels which can lead to excessive appetite.
- depletion of nutrients in '*non*-organic' foods leading to excess grazing through calories to meet minimum nutritional needs.
- diminishing metabolic rate of caloric burn caused by a variety of reasons, including the decline of hormones.
- other causes of excessive appetite and weight gain such as intestinal yeast infection and eating to quiet uncomfortable emotions.
- inadequate physical activity.

One of the more common causes of unwanted weight

gain is the excessive intake of carbohydrates. Because fat deposition is so obvious in extra weight gain, there is a generalized 'fear of fat.' More often, at the root of the problem is excessive intake of carbohydrates.

As you probably know, pure food consists of carbohydrates, proteins, fats, vitamins and minerals. Carbohydrates are comprised, in essence, of long chains of glucose molecules that break down to glucose by a healthy digestive process.

Glucose is like rocket fuel: it burns 'hot' through a process called 'oxidation.' You may know that excessive oxidation can be harmful to the body, which is why you hear so much about "anti-oxidants." (Although there is more to oxidation than just glucose). Glucose is so quick to "oxidize" that it is a far more 'dangerous' molecule, if not carefully managed, than fat (which oxidizes slowly). So, we have exquisite systems to carefully manage glucose.

Our body strongly regulates the amount of glucose available in the blood at any moment and readily converts glucose to safer, slower-to-oxidize fuels: fats. Our physiology aggressively prevents excesses of glucose by a significant protective mechanism that relies upon, among other things, a hormone called insulin. Insulin encourages energy storage. Insulin reduces excessive glucose levels in the blood by causing the glucose to move out of the blood and into cells (see figure 25a on the next page). Interestingly, insulin also causes fats that are in the blood to move into cells.

The process of glucose regulation begins with diges-

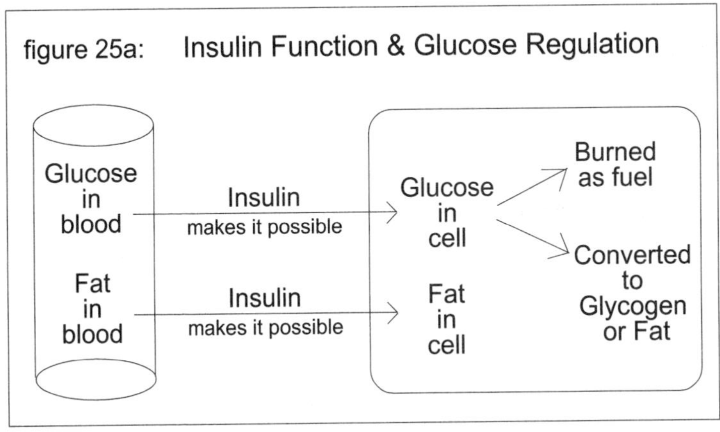

tion. Carbohydrates are digested down to glucose molecules. As soon as glucose is absorbed out of the intestine and into the blood of the 'portal vein' (a blood vessel that goes from the intestine directly to the liver), sensors in the portal vein detect its presence. During a meal that contains carbohydrates, after initial digestion and after breakdown of that carbohydrate to glucose, the absorption of glucose will raise the portal vein glucose content (see figure 25b below) above an acceptable upper limit. The sensors in the

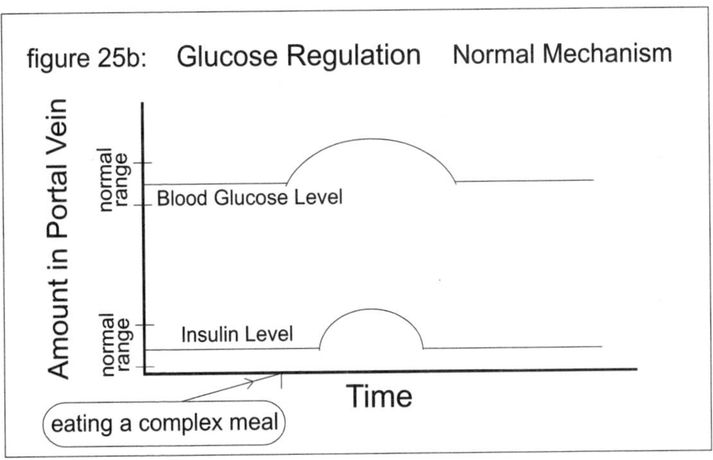

portal vein then call for the release of insulin. Much of the glucose from the meal is, as a result of insulin action, immediately taken up by the liver and other cells. As that occurs, the blood glucose level falls beneath the upper limit of optimal range, thus terminating the need for and the secretion of insulin. Note that the food that is illustrated in figure 25b, has a slow and gradual digestion and absorption rate: it is obviously a more complex food to digest and assimilate.

There is no immediate metabolic need for *all* of the glucose that would be available from a meal that contains abundant carbohydrates. Also, we wouldn't want excessive, easy-to-oxidize glucose floating about with no immediate purpose. Therefore, much of this glucose is taken up by and processed in the liver. There it is converted to

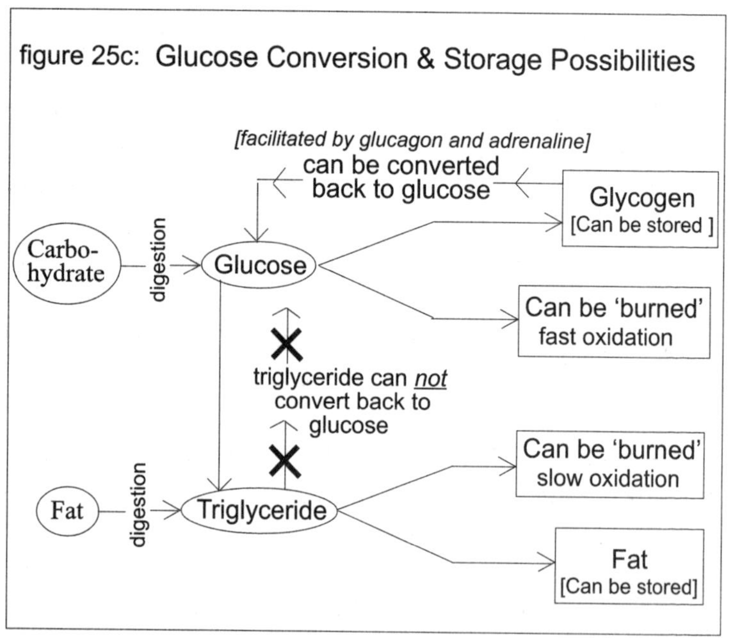

storage forms, either as glycogen, a re-usable form of carbohydrate, or as simple fats called 'triglycerides' or 'cholesterol' (see figure 25c on preceding page).

Important characteristics of and facts related to these conversions include:

- The brain, red blood cells, and certain kidney cells can burn only glucose. All other body cells can burn either glucose or triglycerides.
- Glycogen *can* be converted back to glucose.
- Triglycerides, as mentioned can be distributed to and enter cells, and 'burn' as fuel or stored as fat.
- Triglycerides, once converted *from* glucose, cannot *convert back* to glucose.

Again, fats are slower and 'quiet' in their oxidation and are thus safer to 'burn,' which is why this conversion to fats takes place. Fats also store easily...and abundantly.

The body stores reserves of fuel to be available for the times in the day when we are not eating or digesting. Glycogen is stored in the liver and the muscles, though not in great quantities. Fat is burned or stored, depending on needs generated by basic living and physical activity. It is the excessive storage of fat that sooner or later in our lives becomes our concern. Remember that fat can be produced from glucose, the base of all carbohydrates!

Again, most, but not all, of our cells can burn either glucose or simple fats, such as triglycerides, to produce energy. Triglycerides, even though derived primarily from glucose, cannot be converted back to glucose. It is not possible for your body to pull glucose from stored fat. It can pull that fat back into service as direct fat fuel for many cells. It cannot convert fat back to glucose.

When you don't listen to the words of your mother and you skip your breakfast or other meals, you gradually use up enough blood glucose to decrease it below an acceptable level. This low blood glucose is not tolerable because many crucial body cells, once again, need energy from actual glucose molecules: the brain, red blood cells and certain kidney cells can burn only glucose.

When blood glucose levels fall, mechanisms to restore these levels back to normal will come into play. The first of these mechanisms is the sensation of 'hunger' to motivate you to go forth and eat food. If you do not go forth, the next of these mechanisms is to tap into glycogen reserves and convert glycogen into glucose. This conversion is facilitated by the hormones epinephrine (adrenaline) and glucagon (see figure 25c, page 128). Thus, when you are hungry you secrete adrenaline for assistance.

When glycogen reserves, which are not extensive to begin with, are too low, the body resorts to yet another mechanism to supply glucose from within. A hormone known in general as a "glucocorticoid" is secreted that can actually stimulate the breakdown and conversion of protein into glucose, in a process called "gluconeogenesis" (see figure 25d on the top of the next page).

The principle source of the protein utilized for conversion to glucose is your muscles. Yikes! Under conditions of a need for glucose you will eventually break down your own muscles! You may have thought by skipping that meal

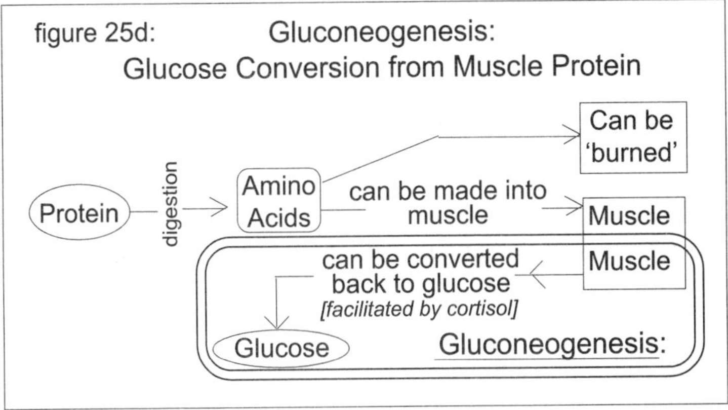

figure 25d: Gluconeogenesis: Glucose Conversion from Muscle Protein

you would lose fat, but in reality what you are losing is muscle.

And by the way, the principle glucocorticoid called upon to initiate gluconeogenesis is named 'cortisol!' By missing meals, and through even more dietary indescretions soon to be described, you can put a strain upon and 'tire out' your cortisol/adrenal mechanisms. You can even adversely affect your immune system with the excess cortisol! Re-

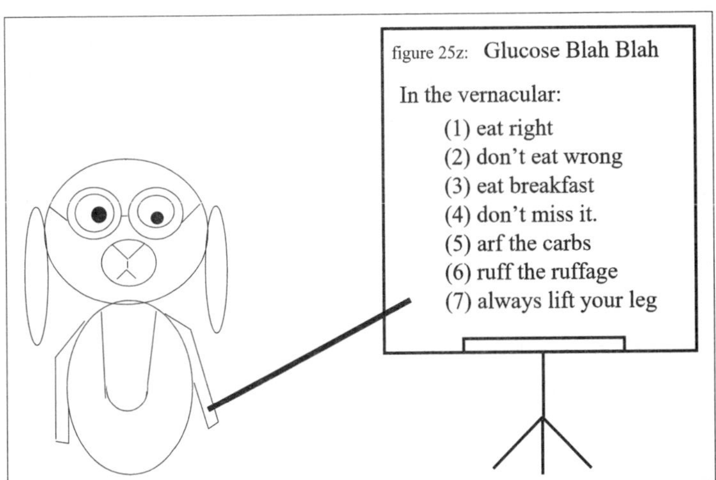

figure 25z: Glucose Blah Blah

markably, we can observe in the sophisticated 24 hour urine hormone test when this particular strain, related to skipped meals (and carbohydrate excess), is being excessively implemented.

Let's focus on this missed breakfast phenomenon in detail. As you can see in figure 25e below, there comes a time after not eating that your blood glucose starts to fall. When it falls beneath an acceptable threshold, you get hungry. If you do not eat, the next step can be that glucose is mobilized from stored glycogen, and eventually, blood glucose is restored to acceptable levels. If the food deprivation goes on too long, you will eventually break down muscle and turn it into glucose, again, by a process that is

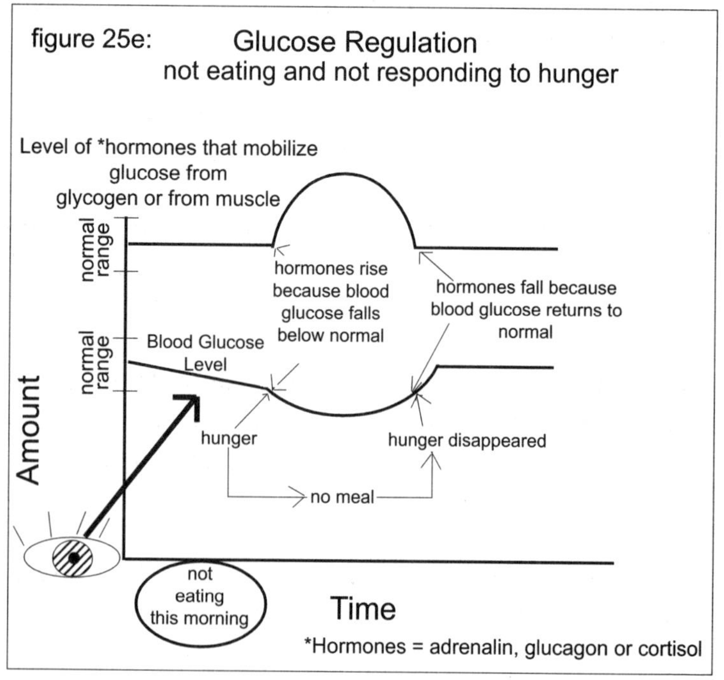

facilitated by a hormone known in general as a 'glucocorticoid,' and specifically as 'cortisol,' in gluconeogenesis.

Have you ever been hungry, not eaten, and noticed that the hunger disappeared? That sensation of hunger occurred because your brain had detected low blood glucose and gave you a strong signal to go out foraging for food. The hunger *disappeared* because when you did not eat, your body secreted adrenaline, glucagon and cortisol, and accessed stored fuel from glycogen, fat, and muscles, as mentioned previously. Once again, it is the cortisol that initiates gluconeogenesis, the conversion of structural protein into glucose. Also, these hormones are appetite suppressive in their own right!

One of the most challenging behaviors to the glucose regulating mechanism is the eating of simple carbohydrates. You know carbohydrates are simple if they are sweet. Look at figure 25f on the next page. Here we see that when you have a sweet, for example a soda pop that has several teaspoons of sugar in it, almost no digestion is required. The sugar is absorbed immediately and blood glucose levels rise very quickly and all at once. Glucose levels go much higher than with complex carbohydrates that digest and assimilate more slowly, over time (see figure 25a). This rapid rise in glucose fools the insulin response. With levels that high your body thinks that you ate a large meal, with more carbohydrates to come, so that you secrete a large amount of insulin. Well, there was no substantial, slower-to-digest complex carbohydrate following the sugar in the soda pop. Your body overestimates. Thus, the excess insulin produces a plummet in the glucose. This plummet (known as 'hypoglycemia'), is unacceptable and once again the adrena-

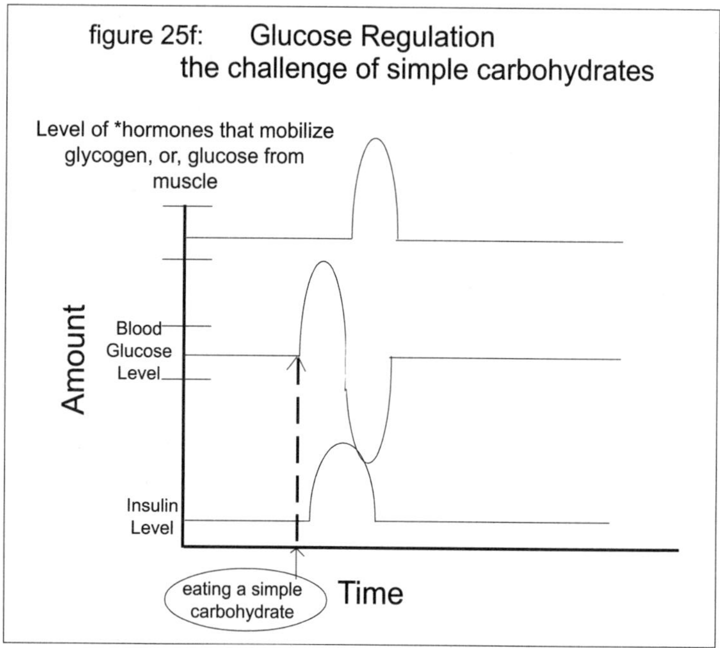

line, glucagon, and glucocorticoids are called into action. This pattern, the taking in of simple carbohydrates, leads to more problems in America than almost any other dietary indescretion!

Do adrenaline and cortisol sound familiar? They are the principal hormonal first-responders in stress. Stress, of course, also has increased metabolic needs, and supplying extra fuel is part of what these stress hormones generate.

Excessive adrenaline and cortisol lead to a biological *insulin resistance*, which is harmful. In this phenomenon, insulin just does not work as well. Often, higher than normal insulin levels are required to overcome this resistance to get the same insulin effect. Another cause of insulin resistance is the long term overstimulation of insulin from *excessive* intake of carbohydrates. As insulin resistance develops, glucose, triglyceride and cholesterol have more difficulty entering cells to be utilized as fuel, and the levels of these elevate in the blood.

The common strategy to lose weight by reducing fats can pose a problem. Fats have acquired such a flawed reputation that the general content of the American diet compared to years ago, has diminished fats... and increased carbohydrates. Many of the carbohydrates will be converted to fat and much of the fat will be stored. Also, if you eat excessive carbohydrates you will have to generate more insulin and thus, raise its levels to higher than ideal. Eventually you will wear down your ability to produce adequate insulin, in the same manner that hormone production is diminished because of long-term overuse in chronic stress. This eventually leads to unbeneficial elevations in blood glucose levels known as 'diabetes.'

Of course there are other factors. Stress raises adrenaline and cortisol levels...and these contribute to insulin resistance. Stimulants such as caffeine and nicotine have the same effect. Look at the possibilities: overeating carbohydrates, skipping meals, and stress all lead to elevated insulin, elevated cortisol and adrenaline, and insulin resistance. When you are no longer young (but still eating as if you were), and become less physically active, the fat deposition begins. So you diet. And you reduce the fat content in your meals because you are afraid of fat. (That means you will emphasize carbohydrates by default). Also, you reduce your calories. But, your brain needs glucose so your adrenaline and cortisol are secreted and you convert your muscles into glucose. Insulin levels rise. You, however, continue to eat carbohydrates. You store more fat!

Because of estrogen, women tend to deposit the fat in the hips and thighs. Because of testosterone, men tend to put it in the abdomen. When women start putting it in the abdomen, we know that insulin resistance has progressed and triglyceride blood levels are increased. Insulin increase causes cholesterol to be dumped into cells. You lose muscle! Wow!

Any discussion of weight gain would be incomplete without mention of the need to reduce calories, choose nutrient rich foods, and address excessive appetite! Calorie strategy for weight loss can be planned with great technical skill: following it and maintaining the weight loss is an art and a strength. You must even be cautious of reducing calories. If you go too far you are liable to start secreting extra adrenaline, etc., to bring blood glucose levels up.

As effective as carefully designed caloric restriction can be it can become very difficult to execute: all of the information I have discussed must be taken into consideration. If, for example, you decide to drop calories by dropping breakfast, you call adrenaline and cortisol into action, fool yourself as they raise blood glucose, suppress appetite, and increase resistance to insulin. By lunch, carbohydrates that you eat will call for insulin in the face of that increased resistance, so higher levels of insulin will be required. This will accelerate fat creation and deposition!

Appetite can be part of the equation for weight reduction. Sometimes appetite is excessive because of:

- habit.
- using food to quiet down emotions or as a substitute for hunger for other things in life.
- diminished neurotransmitters. A topic unto itself. Principle neurotransmitters can diminish over time, by the same mechanism in which stress can cause the overproduction then fatigue of hormones. The most effective (and poisonous!) appetite suppressant, “Phen-fen” contained amphetamine, which is a long-acting artificial adrenaline! Neurotransmitter levels can be tested. Neurotransmitter deficiencies can be addressed with amino acid supplements that are the precursors to them. Consult someone knowledgable in this. When approached incompletely, especially by not identifying or addressing specific deficiencies and creating a balance, results can be unsatisfying. When neurotransmitter repletion is addressed skillfully, successful appetite suppression can result.
- use of non-organic food. Agribusiness food has drastically reduced nutrient content. You can eat a meal that has adequate calories yet contains 15% of the mineral content of organic food. You try to leave the table, yet have cravings for the minerals that were deficient. These cravings actually translate into desire to graze through more food (thus through more calories!) to get what was missing.

As a final consideration, let’s test your strength and endurance by tying all of this in with hormones!

With regard to hormones, metabolism, as I have mentioned before, is dependent upon many factors including thyroid hormone function. Thyroid function is a major determiner of 'rate of burn,' and it is hard to lose weight when you are functionally low in thyroid hormone. Proper thyroid hormone function can itself be dependent upon adequate progesterone levels. Once again, we see the importance of hormones and the importance of progesterone.

Insulin affects hormones. It causes an increase in androgens. This can affect ovulation in young women. Egg development depends on the binding of estradiol to the cell surface of the maturing ovum. Increased androgens can interfere with that binding, block maturation and the needed LH surge, and thus, interfere with ovulation. No ovulation results in greatly diminished progesterone. Diminishing insulin through insulin-lowering choices can restore normal periods in a younger woman.

Estrogens enhance insulin sensitivity. Diminished estrogen is accompanied by diminished insulin sensitivity. Follow that thought as it ties in to menopause and weight.

Testosterone increases insulin resistance. Birth control pills have an artificial progesterone in them ("progestins") that behave more like testosterone than progesterone. Taking birth control pills to restore or regulate periods in menopause can be plenty problematic for weight.

If this chapter interests you, I highly recommend the book The Schwartzbein Principle, with companion cookbooks, by Diana Schwartzbein M.D. She is an endocrinologist with an exquisite understanding of this topic.

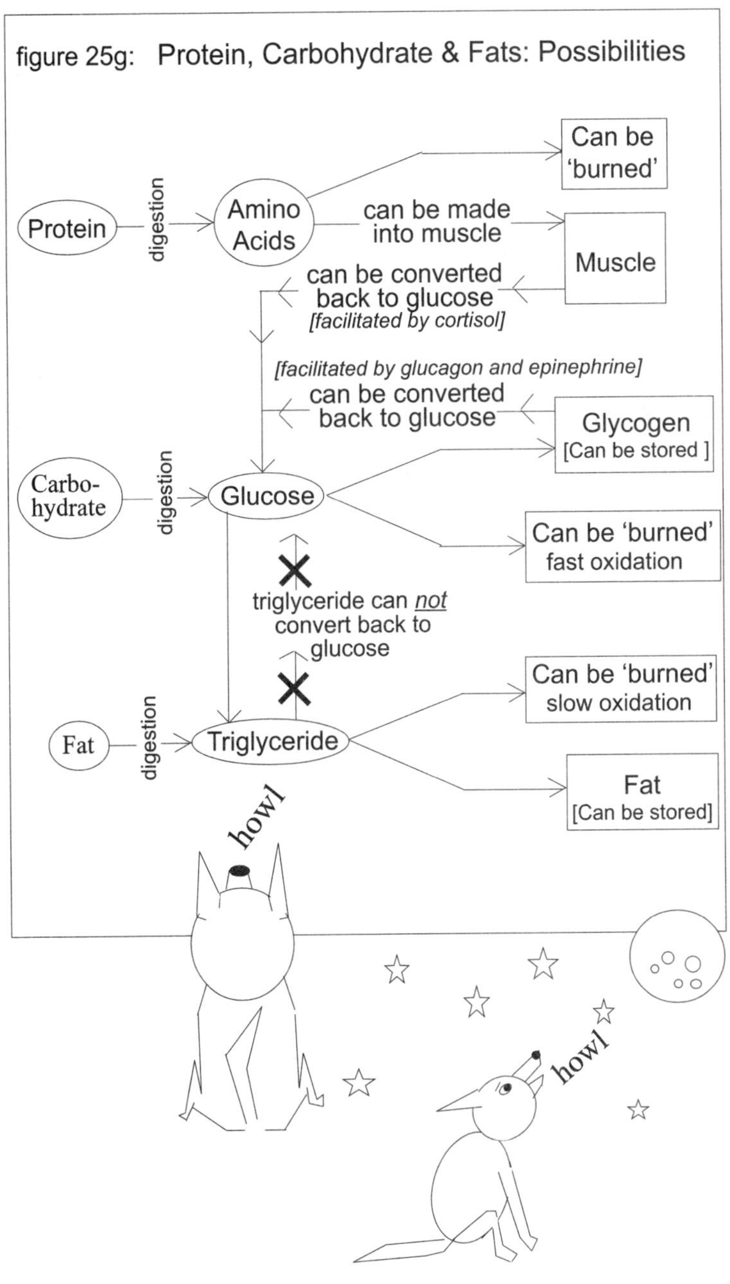
figure 25g: Protein, Carbohydrate & Fats: Possibilities
Protein
digestion
Amino Acids
Can be 'burned'
can be made into muscle
Muscle
can be converted back to glucose
[facilitated by cortisol]
[facilitated by glucagon and epinephrine]
can be converted back to glucose
Glycogen [Can be stored]
Carbo-hydrate
digestion
Glucose
Can be 'burned' fast oxidation
triglyceride can not convert back to glucose
Can be 'burned' slow oxidation
Fat
digestion
Triglyceride
Fat [Can be stored]
howl
howl

To summarize weight loss:

- Effort to not call for excessive insulin by reducing carbohydrate intake, stress, stimulants such as caffeine and nicotine, and increasing exercise.

- Eat organic, so that the food you do eat has the maximum amount of nutrients available and does not leave you hungry to graze through more calories.

- Assess, address and balance hormones.

- Carefully consider a sophisticated calorie reduction program.

- Graze throughout the day, not missing meals or snacks.

- Take a good multivitamin and mineral, and perhaps other specific nutritional supplements needed in reduced caloric eating.

- Eat whole foods and minimize processed foods.

- Optimize your digestion and absorption by chewing as well as considering supplementing with digestive enzymes and even hydrochloric acid.

- Investigate and address neurotransmitter repletion for better ease with appetite issues.

Chapter Fourteen

Menopause: An Opportunity to Become More

by Lyn Marsh Ph.D.

Menopause can feel like a horror. Menopause can also inspire positive changes in your life. Many women are afraid to face menopause because they feel that they are going to lose touch with how they have identified themselves. Some are threatened by their approaching inability to have children. Some women are afraid that they will no longer be as sexually attractive, and therefore they could lose love, or maybe never find love again.

This is understandable when you look at how our society defines sexual attractiveness. Being sexually attractive infers that you look like what they display in the media. Women are mostly presented as objects of seduction, with limited, and always very young, body shapes.

In the process of trying to live up to, or even push up against, these constrained and limited views of what being attractive means, women have lost some of their truer meaning in life. If this truer meaning is lost, then to approach menopause can be a horror. It can feel like a horrendous loss.

This loss is felt so intensely when there is nothing of greater meaning to replace how you have identified yourself. There is so much more to life, than what size you are, or how many wrinkles you have, or how much you sag. There is more to life than raising children, even though this can be a fulfilling and rewarding era. What follows can be more, more than you expect or even hope for.

In order to transform this journey of menopause from a potential horror into an adventure that inspires you to transcend your very image and identity of who you are, you need to look beyond what society offers you.

It is possible to transmute and transform menopause into a time of miraculous growth. Hormones have sometimes driven your body, driven your mind, and even driven you mad. These hormones are slowing down. Your drives, your needs, and your desires are changing. Who are you now? Who are you becoming?

When you enter into menopause, so many identities that you have of yourself can come to the surface for re-examination. Your old identities may not seem to work as well for you any more.

Who are you now? Who are you becoming?

Throughout your life you have become at least somewhat familiar with your creativity and with your nurturing capacities. It is more of the knowing and the wisdom that awaits you now. But before you will allow yourself to become more wise, you need to face where and who you are in your life now. This is necessary before you will allow the wisdom to guide you into a life that is abounding with the love you so want to know, with passion and a vibrancy, with creativity and imagination that fill your world.

If you are willing to face your self, and face what and who you are now, then you can begin to move beyond your current way of experiencing life, into a life that can express more of who you really are. And this life is going to be much more fulfilling than your current life, no matter how fulfilled you are now. From here, you can reach into an ancient knowing and wisdom that can illuminate through you, from seemingly out of nowhere.

Many women recoil here, because they think that if they focus on this potential knowing and wisdom, they will lose their creativity or their passion, or have to give up their nurturing. They are afraid that they will lose their sexual appeal. They are terrified of losing the love.

You can reach into an ancient knowing and wisdom that can illuminate through you, from seemingly out of nowhere.

There are so many limited images and beliefs that separate wisdom and knowing from love, passion, and vibrancy. You see these images of old old men and women barely hobbling around with canes, with zero passion and dried up expressions. Well, these are the personifications of the bleached out views that try to wipe out the richness and depth of what living a life replete with knowing and wisdom is about!

Wisdom and knowing actually flow from a deep passion, a sensuousness, and a deep sensuality within life. Wisdom and knowing flow out of a romance, a romance at the deepest level, with life itself. Wisdom and knowing flow out of love, out of a loving that has no words.

You will not lose your connection with loving, passion, or romance, if you allow your wisdom and knowing to flow.

You can actually access passion and romance in ways that you never knew existed. And this will not be written about in the media. You can find new ways of loving and being loved, ways that can lift you into a renewed peace and joy, into a beauty that changes your life. You can access power that will knock your socks off!

Some women who reach this stage of growing and changing, get confused. They can become misdirected because they are beginning to look deeper, yet they don't have

Wisdom and knowing actually flow from a deep passion, a sensuousness, and a deep sensuality within life. Wisdom and knowing flow from a romance with life itself. Wisdom and knowing flow out of a loving that has no words.

a solid artistry or mastery developed with being more wise and knowing. They may be courageous enough to begin to see more of the truth of what is not working in their relationships, for example. And as they first wake up to this, they can assess that the way to change is to throw out their current life. They may leave their partners or impulsively quit their jobs and leap out into the void with a re-found, but misdirected passion. They may think that by doing this, they can go find that love or passion, that is out in that world somewhere.

This is not a necessary or helpful direction, to make the

changes you desire. The love and passion, the wisdom and knowing are actually within you. It is more about finding these within the more real that you are, and from here you allow more love, healing, and joy into your life. It all flows the opposite way that society portrays it.

There are times, when leaving a relationship or a work situation will support you in your life. But these decisions and choices are best made, outside of the heat that menopause can produce. This is not to infer that you should stay in a destructive relationship or work situation until you have gone through menopause, because, that will not work. Rather, it seems more productive, to do your work with yourself, then go back and look at the changes that you want to make. And make them from a place of empowerment within you. This way you can make these decisions and choices from a knowing inside of you, instead of an instantaneous heated reaction to a chronic situation.

You can develop a trust with yourself by following your heart and your mind. Along with this, you can open yourself up to your deeper feelings and emotions. Then, with compassion for yourself and your life, you can make your choices from the greater understanding and knowing that emerge from this self-discovery.

Becoming more of who you are capable of being, is not about blaming or punishing others for your upset. It is about taking responsibility for your life, as it is now, and from here, making choices and decisions that inspire you to become more of who you are capable of being.

And, who you are capable of being, is what is left, when

you let go of who you are not.

Blaming yourself or another, is who you are not,. Negatively judging yourself or others, is also who you are not. Feeling sorry for yourself, is who you are not. Feeling burdened by life, or by others' expectation of you, is who you are not. Feeling weak and trying to get others to be strong for you, is who you are not. Feeling like you can not change your life, and having a list of reasons about why this is true, is who you are not.

As you let go of these beliefs and ways of being, who you are becoming will begin to flow. Who you are becoming can not be defined in ways with which you are familiar. It is important to let this be a mystery to you. This mystery of you can then find its way into your life and into your very being, within your life.

How Do You Currently Identify Yourself?

Are you a creative, nurturing, giving person? Do you consider yourself to be self-focused and less interested in the needs of others? Do you see your self to be achievement oriented? Do you consider yourself to be a good friend? Or are you a mediocre friend to others? Do you feel that you are a happy person or a sad or a disappointed or lonely person? Do you feel that you are being pulled from every direction? Do you feel that you are being ignored or put

And, who you are capable of being, is what is left, when you let go of who you are not.

down? Or do you feel content in your life?

When you enter into menopause, all of these identities that you have of yourself, and so many more issues, may come to the surface for re-examination.

Now Is A Grand Time To Heal

You can move beyond the limited definitions and identities that you have used to make up your current image of yourself. This image may have gotten you what you thought you wanted, in the past, but it probably does not work well now! It is unlikely that you want the same things now. You need a new image. In fact, the old one will eventually take you down, if you don't put it down.

You can begin to remember why you are alive at all. The knowing and wisdom can begin to take you forward into a new arena of living. Here you are empowered to bring more happiness and more fulfillment to your life.

How Do You Reach Into This Knowing And Wisdom?

You can begin this process, by facing where your life is now. What have you been avoiding about yourself or your life? Look into this from both the negative and positive perspectives.

What in your life has been hurting you that you haven't wanted to see or admit? What or who have you been hurting in your life that you have been afraid to admit? What do you have rage about? What is really behind that chronic de-

Now Is A Grand Time To Heal

pression you have been feeling? What have you been secretly feeling, that you don't feel like you have had permission to feel, or at least, to feel directly and openly?

In order to face and reveal some of the answers to these, and other, questions, you must let go of your automatic and harmful judgments of yourself. You may be making judgments about your body, or about how you are never good enough. You may be telling yourself that you are less than or better than others. You may be telling yourself that you don't deserve to have what matters to you.

What in your life has been hurting you that you haven't wanted to see or admit?

More than ever, you now need to have compassion for who you are, for all of your failures and mistakes, and for how you have failed yourself. Answering the questions above only becomes possible as you are willing to have compassion. If you hold on to those destructive judgments of yourself, you will use some of what you discover, to punish and hurt yourself more. And if you continue to do this, you will not be willing to change. And the cycle of self-destructive behaviors would keep going around and around.

As you face yourself, with compassion, while acknowledging and taking responsibility for the negative impact that you have had on others and for the negative impact that you have allowed others to have upon you, from here, you can forgive yourself. When you forgive, you open yourself to what is beyond your failures, your disappointments, and your suffering. You open yourself to that deeper knowing and wisdom that will then come to you.

When you are willing to forgive yourself, you can change your life. You will not be willing to truly change your life until you are willing to forgive.

At this point, all you have to do, to begin receiving more of the wisdom and knowing available to you, is to close your eyes and ask for greater understanding and knowing in your life:

> Imagine that there is a very wise and ancient person standing in front of you. You may not feel that this person is real, but, as you imagine this ancient one next to you, you are communicating your desire for more knowing and wisdom. And this will open a portal so that more wisdom and knowing can be received by you.

> If You Open, It Will Come To You

> You may ask this ancient one for more understanding, knowing, and/or wisdom within your life as a whole, or you may have particular areas of concern that you want deeper understanding and knowing about.

> After you ask, thank them, and then let go of your focus, pause, and go about other activities in your life. Then, later, you may

> have insights that come to you from out of nowhere, or you may see a book on the shelf that stands out to you, that will contain the knowing that you desire. You may have a friend tell you what you need to hear. Or a movie on TV may give you a message that wakes something up in you.

Greater knowing and wisdom can also be available through the avenues of admitting the good, the true, and the beautiful about your self. This admitting is actually much harder than you might at first think! We recoil from seeing what we judge as negative about ourselves, yet the exquisite beauty of who we are, is even more threatening to us! It is so very important to look deeper into your life, to see the beauty of how you love, and of how you give.

You can look at how you have helped another feel happier or more confident. How have you helped others express more of their strengths and power? How have you loved so that others have felt more love in their life? How have you inspired others? How have you brought more beauty into the life of others? How have you helped another resolve something that felt impossible to them?

Greater knowing and wisdom can also be available through the avenues of admitting the good, the true, and the beautiful about your self

Some Things to Remember

Life is so very much more than we have known it to be. Life is a dream. As you begin to let the possibility of this affect you, everything in life begins to become more alive. You begin to live your life with grace.

Living your life with more grace can inspire you to change what drives you within your life. The greatest drive that exists, is to unveil or unravel the secrets and mysteries of life and of love. You can unravel the mysteries about who you are and about how you want to express yourself in this world. You can begin allowing yourself to be driven by unraveling the mysteries of what love is really about.

You can also begin to allow yourself fulfillment of your greatest need, that of being truly loving, (instead of trying to get someone to love you). You can find fulfillment of your greatest desire: to be happy, to have more joy in your life.

The greatest drive that exists, is to unveil or unravel the secrets and mysteries of life and of love

You are so much more than you acknowledge and know. For the rest of your life, you could find out more and more about what that statement means. You could search forever and this would be only the beginning, a beginning with no end, an eternal discovery of who you are. A journey where every moment is filled more and more,

You can fulfill your greatest need, that of being truly loving

with all that you are and all that you can be. Where every moment is eternal. Here you can brush across the knowing that you are eternal. As you begin to let this knowing change you, everything changes. Everything becomes more alive with the mystery, the mystical, and the magical of what life can be. *

Everything becomes more alive
with the mystery,
the mystical,
and the magical
of what life can be

** Lyn Marsh Ph.D. attributes her success and much of the influence in her writing to Lazaris' teachings. Lazaris teaches about creating success in your reality. She feels deep gratitude for Lazaris and for Lazaris' immense love and guidance. She feels deep appreciation and thanks for Concept Synergy. The writings of Lyn Marsh do not necessarily reflect the teachings of Lazaris or Concept Synergy.*

Chapter Fifteen

Grand Summary

We have been on a long journey together, and it has been exciting one. Let me summarize what we have been considering.

Each woman entering, or, in menopause, differs in

- individual vigor of health
- number and significance of health issues
- sensitivity to treatments
- biologic individuality
- fundamental ovarian and overall hormonal balance
- and, risk factors for disease.

Treating menopause elegantly can involve:

- Careful assessment of the above issues through a medical and hormonal history and a physical examination.

- Further evaluation by hormonal and other testing when indicated.

- Treatment by carefully selected bio-identical hormones, most often in the form of hydroalcoholic skin gels.

- Adjustment of programs, especially titrating the hormonal dosage levels in accord with symptoms of insufficiency or excess.

- Attention to the liver, intestine and other systems when indicated, especially if there are symptoms of, or risk factors for, female organ illnesses and when estrogens are used in treatment.

- Supplementation with additional Folic acid, Vitamin B6, sublingual Vitamin B12, and Indole-3-carbinol for the beneficial effects they have on the biochemical processing of estrogens.

- Attention to the issue of osteoporosis through consideration of diet, digestion, and absorption, hormones, supplementation, and the possibility of excessive acidity.

- Consumption of organic, whole, non-processed food as much as possible. For many, reduce carbohydrates and all-but-eliminate simple carbohydrates.

- Awareness of and attention to the emotions, consciousness, life, love and dreams in all women and men.

At first it may seem like a lot to do, yet as you do it, you will get good at it. It may become second nature to you and can serve you well for many years.

To summarize weight loss:

- Effort to not call for excessive insulin by reducing carbohydrate intake, stress, stimulants such as caffeine and nicotine, and increasing exercise.

- Eat oganic, so that the food you do eat has the maximum amount of nutrients available and does not leave you hungry to graze through more calories.

- Address and balance hormones.

- Carefully consider a sophisticated calorie reduction program.

- Graze throughout the day, not missing meals or snacks.

- Take a good multivitamin and mineral, and perhaps other specific nutritional supplements.

- Eat whole foods and minimize processed foods.

- Optimize your digestion and absorption by chewing as well as considering supplementing with digestive enzymes and even hydrochloric acid.

- Investigate and address neurotransmitters for better ease in appetite issues.

On the next four pages, you will find summary charts of hormone gel application.

figure 26a: **Skin Gels in General:**

Apply before bedtime and in the morning
Exception:
You may find that you can do just as well with one application of gels per day, for convenience

Apply starting with feet & ankles, then legs, then knees and thighs, etc until you reach 'the top' [your forehead]...then begin again
Exception:
save a little for your face, neck & back of hands every time
Exception:
Do not apply estrogens to the front of your torso [neck to pubic area, and between your shoulders]
Exception:
Do not apply testosterone to the front of your torso or to face or to hairy areas of your body

---

figure 26b: **Finding Optimal Dose of Progesterone by Symptoms of Inadequacy and Excess**

Progesterone deficiency:

sleep problems
breast tenderness
water retention
emotional mood problems, sometimes severe
period irregularities if you are still menstruating

Adequate Progesterone:

Improved sleep
Reduced breast tenderness
Feeling more relaxed, in better mood
Decreased water retention
A more regular period if you are still menstruating

Progesterone Excess

Drowsiness
Waking up groggy or edgy
Slight dizziness
Increased water retention
Sense of physical instability
Depressed feeling
Feeling of being drunk or spinning
Heaviness of the extremities

Unusual Response to Progesterone

Antsy, anxious, can't sleep & water retention [cortisol & deoxycorticosterone are related to the cause]
Hot flashes, or depression [overload of estrogen receptors]
Increased appetite + weight gain [unclear cause]
[Possible increased incidence of Candida Albicans]

figure 26c: Progesterone: Treatment Summary

Progesterone gel 3% 30 mg/g 1 gram = 1/4 tsp
Progesterone capsules 50 or 100 mg strength,
50 - 150 mg additional progesterone
may be needed at night
Progesterone gel 10% sometimes used when
greater amounts of progesterone are needed
Administration in menopause:
1/8th to 1/4 tsp 1 or 2 times daily.
possibly more or all at night
possibly additional progesterone in capsule form
for help with sleep disturbance
Administration in perimenopause:
administer in 2nd half of cycle
possibly administer during first half of cycle,
from day 5 to 13
stop taking before your anticipated period
[example: day 28]

- Spotting occasionally when your cycle remains regular can be acceptable. Disregard the spotting and continue taking progesterone. This should regulate you. If it does not, consult your physician.
- Should an unusually heavy flow occur, stop progesterone and consider this day of heavy flow to be the first day of your period. Resume progesterone 5 or 14 days later, according to previous guidelines.
- If your period does not come after stopping progesterone, designate the day you stopped as the first day of your cycle. Start progesterone again in 5 or 14 days.
- At times estrogen dominant symptoms may not be ameliorated after reasonable effort. For one possibility, your liver may not be metabolizing estrogens properly or adequately. In this case estrogen levels build up. Sometimes it is necessary to take measures beyond treatment with progesterone, such as addressing liver function and detoxification.
- Some women do poorly on progesterone! It may not make sense, yet they do not like progesterone at all.

figure 26d: Finding Optimal Dose of Hormones by Symptoms of Inadequacy and Excess

Estrogen

Inadequate:

Hot flashes
Vaginal dryness
Loss of breast fullness, drooping
Sleep disturbance: difficulty falling asleep, with restlessness, night sweats
Mind foggy in the morning,
Feeling a "little down"
Confused, not in good control of your mood

Excess:

Breast tenderness, especially in nipple area
Water retention, rings too tight
Feeling uptight, irritated, yet with a clear mind
Breast fullness, growing

figure 26e: Estrogen Treatment Summary

Bi-est Gel:
Do not apply to the front of the torso
2.75 mg/gram = 0.75 mg/g Estradiol [E2], 2 mg/g Estriol [E3]
1/8th tsp = 0.5 gram, 1/4 tsp = 1 gram
Common starting dose: Apply 1/8th tsp 1 or 2 times/day increase dosages by 1/16th tsp [1/2 of 1/8th tsp] if necessary
If you have night sweats, increase the night dose.
Adjust, adjust, adjust!
If menstruating, begin on day 5, end on day 28, and follow the 'estrogen menstrual curve' [figure 2]

figure 26f: Finding Optimal Dose of Hormones by Symptoms of Inadequacy and Excess

Testosterone

Inadequate:

Diminished libido
Loss of sense of security
Diminished energy and stamina
Flabbiness & Muscular weakness;
upper arms, cheeks
Hair loss

Excess:

Hyper aggressiveness
Hair growth in unwanted places
face, and where gel is applied
Acne
Excessive oiliness of skin

Figures & Charts

Figures & Charts, continued

Index

C

D

E

F

I

K

L

M

N

O

P

R

S

V

W

Notes

Notes

Menopause is at the boundary of
your new frontier.

Menopause can be a time for
valuing yourself and
knowing the significance of who you are.

You can come to love yourself
more than you have dreamed.

You can lift yourself
out of your limitations.

Your soul communicates with you through the
language of
imagination and your dreams.
And your soul is the window to the
divine.

You can unveil the love that you truly are,
realize the dreams that
your soul and spirit have for you,
and
dream the dreams
that you never knew you had.

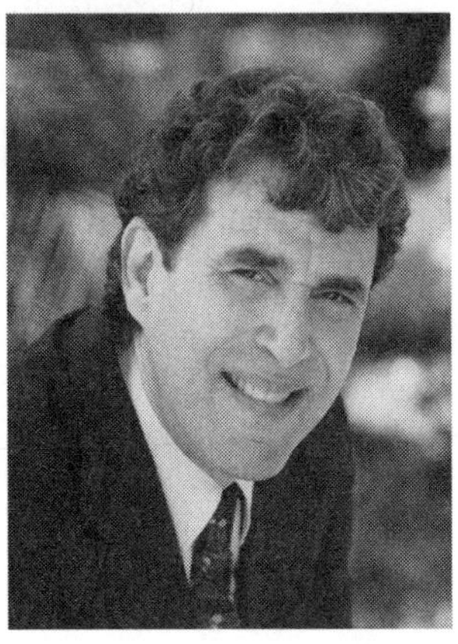

Daved Rosensweet M.D.

Dr. Rosensweet graduated from the University of Michigan Medical School in 1968. While his knowledge is based in traditional training, he uses methods which he learned from renown pioneers and practitioners in the Holistic field. He has been in private Holistic medical practice since 1971, and has had offices in New Mexico, California, and Colorado. Early in his career he delivered over 300 babies at home. He has been in charge of health promotion for the State of New Mexico, has lectured widely, has taught Holistic Medicine to physicians and the public, has hosted and produced "Get Well: Stay Well" a TV show on health, and guides an ongoing seminar, "The Healing Process."

He currently is a medical associate at the Perlmutter Health Center in Naples Florida as well as in private practice in Sarasota Florida. He lives with his wife Lyn, and their four animals, Sparkle, Wonder, Magic Carlos and Star.